Corneal Surgery

Bruno Zuberbuhler • Stephen Tuft
David Gartry • David Spokes

Corneal Surgery

Essential Techniques

Springer

Authors
Bruno Zuberbuhler
Ophthalmology, St. Thomas' Hospital
London
United Kingdom

David Gartry
Moorfields Eye Hospital
London
United Kingdom

Stephen Tuft
Moorfields Eye Hospital
London
United Kingdom

David Spokes
St. James's University Hospital
Leeds
United Kingdom

Illustrator
Reinhold Henkel
Heidelberg
Germany

Additional material to this book can be downloaded from http://extras.springer.com

ISBN 978-3-662-50579-3 ISBN 978-3-642-12502-7 (eBook)
DOI 10.1007/978-3-642-12502-7
Springer Heidelberg New York Dordrecht London

Softcover reprint of the hardcover 1st edition 2013

Printed on acid-free paper

Springer is part of Springer Science+Business Media (www.springer.com)

Preface

This book has been written for those who manage patients with corneal and external eye disease and who are looking for instant access to detailed clinical information. It brings together the advantage of a handbook, high quality images, easy-to-understand illustrations and a collection of the most common surgical procedures on video.

The aspiration of this book has been for it to be a portable repository of knowledge, accessible in eye casualty, corneal clinic and theatre instantly. Although it covers the whole range of corneal surgery, including refractive laser surgery techniques, this book is not exhaustive and we would like it to complement the existing series of desktop ophthalmology heavyweights.

Our aim is to focus on the integration of evidence-based and established treatment options rather than the presentation of cutting edge new procedures that might not be widely available to the readers.

Another element of this book is to provide tips and tricks for wet lab based self-learning techniques. We believe that surgery as a 'manual art' has to be practised outside the theatre as often as possible to increase the dexterity and to be able to provide the efficiency and accuracy needed to fulfil patients' high outcome expectations, in particular in refractive laser eye surgery.

It is hoped that this first edition will not be the last, and we welcome any comments and suggestions from junior and senior readers that will help us to make future editions even better.

London, UK — Bruno Zuberbuhler
London, UK — Stephen Tuft
London, UK — David Gartry
Leeds, UK — David Spokes

Acknowledgements

We would like to thank the many Ophthalmologists who supported this book. We especially thank the senior corneal surgeons who generously contributed video footage, including Francisco Arnalich from the Hospital Universitario Ramón y Cajal, Madrid, Spain; Andrew Morrell and James Ball from St James's University Hospital, Leeds, United Kingdom.

It has been a great pleasure to work with Alan Lacey from W3 Media Ltd on the DVD production. We would like to thank Abbott and Alcon for images and support with the DVD.

I am grateful to all the team at Springer, including Irmela Bohn, Sabine Ehlenbeck, Sverre Klemp and Rosemarie Unger. Thanks to Reinhold Henkel who created beautiful medical illustrations.

BZ would like to thank Kasia and Helena for their inspiration and patience.

Contents

Introduction

1

1.1 Development of Corneal Surgery

1.1.1 Brief History of Corneal Transplantation

The idea of restoring clarity to an opaque cornea has existed for far longer than the means to achieve it has been available. During the late nineteenth century, various xenografts were attempted between animal species, all unsuccessful. In 1905, Zirm performed the first successful human penetrating keratoplasty (PKP) and thus the first successful human organ allograft. The enucleated eyes of an 11-year-old boy with intraocular foreign bodies provided healthy corneas that were transplanted into a recipient blinded by a previous alkali injury. Remarkably, in this pre-antibiotic, pre-corticosteroid era, one graft survived and provided the patient with useful vision.

Further work by Castroviejo and Filatov (among others) enabled the subsequent development of PKP from a procedure of last resort to one of routine clinical practice. This was facilitated by the development of operating microscopes, improvements in instrumentation and sutures, understanding of immune modulation and the development of topical corticosteroids, and advances in optimal preservation of tissue between retrieval and transplantation.

Lamellar surgery as a concept predates penetrating keratoplasty, but universally early efforts resulted in opacity. In the modern era the development of techniques by Barraquer, Melles and Anwar has enabled successful selective tissue replacement with proven advantages over PKP.

Affected epithelium or stroma can be replaced by deep anterior lamellar keratoplasty (DALK) which preserves the host Descemet's membrane (DM) and endothelium. Melles' innovation was to use air in the anterior chamber to create a light reflex to guide sharp dissection as close to DM as possible. Anwar used injection of an air bubble to create a cleavage plane between stroma and DM.

Posterior lamellar surgery has evolved in recent years under the influence of Melles and Terry. Deep lamellar endothelial keratoplasty (DLEK) involves dissecting out a disc of posterior stroma bearing DM and endothelium and replacing it with a similar portion of donor tissue. Melles subsequently established that excision of the host posterior stroma was not necessary and that donor stroma bearing DM and endothelium could be applied after stripping DM and endothelium from the host cornea, a procedure termed Descemet's stripping with endothelial keratoplasty (DSEK).

Descemet's membrane endothelial keratoplasty (DMEK) is the latest refinement of the technique, wherein only DM and endothelium are implanted. Further details of all these techniques can be found in later sections of this book.

1.1.2 Brief History of Refractive Laser Surgery

The excimer laser (*EXCI*ted di*MER*) was introduced in industry in the late 1970s for the manufacture of printed circuit boards. During

B. Zuberbuhler et al., *Corneal Surgery*,
DOI 10.1007/978-3-642-12502-7_1, © Springer-Verlag Berlin Heidelberg 2013

the early 1980s Srinivasan at IBM noted that it could be used to sculpt biological tissues to sub-micrometer precision with no thermal damage to surrounding tissue. The laser beam is in the ultraviolet (UV) range (193 nm for ArF laser) and is therefore of very high energy and low penetration into tissues. Absorption of laser results in release of energy sufficient to disrupt molecular bonds in tissues, resulting in ablation of the target. The development of computers to direct the beam and control the profile of tissue reshaping facilitated the introduction of excimer lasers in ophthalmology.

Excimer lasers were first used to produce radial keratotomies but soon abandoned in favour of surface ablations. Phototherapeutic keratectomy (PTK) was the first application, which involves the removal of abnormal superficial corneal tissue. Careful design of the ablation profile allows refractive errors to be corrected (photorefractive keratotomy, PRK), but this is painful and the healing response may cause haze. Performing the ablation on stroma after reflecting a superficial flap allowed correction of refractive error and avoided the discomfort and haze of surface treatments. This is termed LASIK (laser-assisted in situ keratomileusis).

The microkeratome necessary for creation of the LASIK flap is based on the invention by Barraquer in the 1950s. In his technique, a 300 μm lamella of cornea was removed, shaped on a cryolathe, and replaced. This was difficult to master and was replaced by in situ sculpting of the cornea (keratomileusis) by two passes of the microkeratome. Evolution of the microkeratome has led to models that are safe and reliable and which cut a hinged flap that can be reflected to expose the stromal bed for ablation by the excimer laser. The latest evolutionary step in LASIK has been the use of femtosecond lasers to create the corneal flap. This avoids much of the unpredictability inherent with mechanical devices and enables the surgeon to create a flap of optimum thickness and profile.

Major events in excimer refractive surgery are shown in Table 1.1.

Table 1.1 Major events in excimer refractive surgery

Year	Author/development
1983	Trokel: excimer laser to reshape cornea
1985	Seiler: first excimer PTK in a sighted eye
1987	McDonald: PRK leading to accidental improvement of vision during a trial on 'blind' eyes
1988	McDonald: FDA trial of PRK
1990	Pallikaris and Burratto: LASIK
1991	First clinical trial of LASIK
1995	FDA approval for PRK
1999	FDA approval for LASIK

1.2 Anatomy of the Cornea and Conjunctiva

1.2.1 Corneal Structures

The cornea begins to develop in utero at around day 33 and continues to mature through to the fifth month. Epithelium is derived from surface ectoderm. The endothelium is derived from mesenchymal cells migrating under the primitive epithelium, and the stroma derives from a later influx of mesenchyme between these two layers. Both endothelium and stroma are of neural crest origin.

A standardised cornea (Fig. 1.1) is 10.6 mm in its vertical meridian and 11.7 mm horizontally. When viewed from the back, however, it is circular. The cornea is prolate aspheric with the central portion having a smaller radius of curvature (7.8 mm) than the periphery. Central corneal thickness is 550 μm increasing to 670 μm at the periphery.

1.2.1.1 Epithelium

The air-tear film interface of the external surface of the cornea is responsible for the greater part of the refractive power of the cornea (and hence that of the entire eye). The corneal epithelium is a stratified squamous non-keratinised layer of 5 or 6 cells thick (50–60 μm). Adjacent cells are bound to each other by desmosomes. Cells of the basal layer are columnar and are bound via

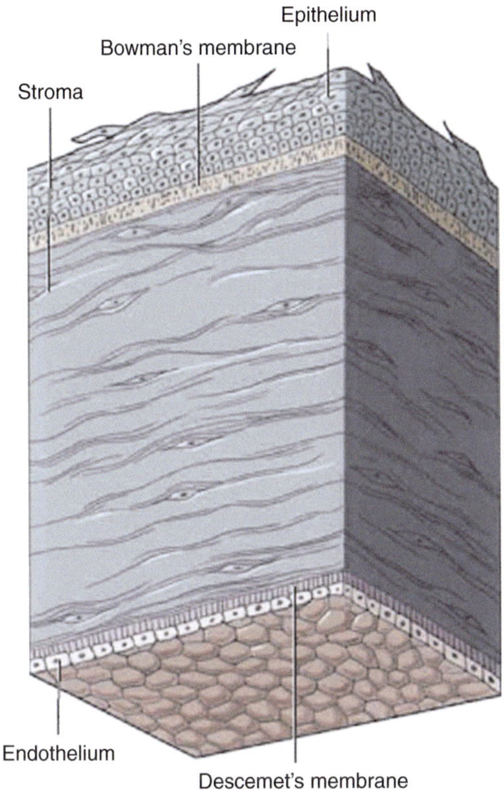

Fig. 1.1 Illustration of corneal anatomy

hemidesmosomes to the underlying basal lamina. Cell division in this layer produces new cells that migrate centripetally and superficially to replace lost or dead cells. Cells become squamous and anuclear as they migrate superficially and are shed into the tear film after a few days.

The external surfaces of superficial epithelial cells have microvilli and microplicae which aid attachment of the mucin layer of the tear film. In some respects the epithelium acts like a fluid to fill in irregularities in the stroma to compensate for small variations in corneal contour.

When injured, the epithelium heals rapidly by cell migration and replication. The central corneal epithelium has no melanocytes or immunocompetent cells, which, along with the absence of blood vessels, contribute to its relative immunological privilege, an important benefit in corneal transplantation.

The basal lamina of the epithelium comprises the lamina lucida (25 nm) and lamina densa (50 nm). Adhesion of the epithelium is achieved via anchoring complexes of collagen that connect it to the lamina densa and Bowman's layer.

1.2.1.2 Bowman's Layer

This is an 8–12 μm thick layer of modified acellular stroma clearly distinct from the basement membrane of the epithelium. Its collagen fibrils are relatively thin and regularly arranged.

1.2.1.3 Stroma

This constitutes 90 % of the thickness of the cornea (450–500 μm) and has a vital role in maintaining the strength and integrity of the cornea. The anterior stroma has the highest tensile strength, with the posterior stroma adjacent to Descemet's membrane being the weakest. It comprises regularly arranged 2 μm thick lamellae collagen fibres, between which are scattered flattened modified fibroblasts termed keratocytes. The regularity of fibril arrangement and spacing between fibrils maintains the transparency of the cornea. At the periphery collagen fibres blend with sclera. The healthy stroma is avascular and without lymphatics. Sensory nerves traverse the stroma from the periphery en route to the epithelium.

1.2.1.4 Descemet's Membrane

This is the modified basement membrane of the endothelium and is 8–12 μm thick. It comprises an anterior banded zone (1/3 of the thickness) that is laid down in utero and a posterior non-banded zone which is deposited throughout life. DM is continuous peripherally with the trabecular meshwork.

1.2.1.5 Endothelium

A monolayer of hexagonal cells 5–6 μm in height and 20 μm in diameter, this layer maintains the cornea in a state of relative dehydration. Adjacent cells are connected via tight junctions. Ion channels in the apical surface actively transport water out of the cornea into the anterior camber to maintain corneal transparency. Endothelial cell densities are 3,000–4,000/mm^2 at birth, and as these cells are not replaced, their numbers fall with age to a density of 2,000/mm^2 in later years. A cell density of less than approximately 800/mm^2 is insufficient to sustain adequate fluid transport, and the cornea becomes oedematous.

1.2.2 Corneal Innervation

The cornea is innervated mainly via the long ciliary nerves derived from the ophthalmic division of the trigeminal nerve. Branches form an annular plexus in the anterior stroma before losing their myelin sheaths and forming a sub-epithelial plexus. This is most dense in the mid-periphery and absent in the central cornea. Further branches then course superficially and centripetally to form a terminal intraepithelial plexus serving pain and temperature (specifically cold) sensation.

1.2.3 Corneal Healing

After injury the epithelium heals by migration of cells adjacent to the traumatised area moving centripetally to completely cover the injured area, in conjunction with division of progenitor cells in the basal layer more peripherally. Movement of cells is regulated by contact inhibition, which prevents over-proliferation and ensures that the final surface is smooth and regular. Division of limbal stem cells produces a population of new epithelial cells that migrate centripetally to continuously replace those lost by shedding or trauma.

An injury to the stroma is repaired by mechanisms that are similar to regeneration in connective tissue generally. Inflammatory cells including macrophages first remove any damaged tissue. New extracellular matrix material is deposited and then remodelled. Activated keratocytes produce collagen to repair the defect, but since this new collagen (types IV and VII) is of a type that is not usually found in stroma (types I and III), and is not laid down in the same ordered fashion, it forms an opaque scar. Subsequent remodelling of this tissue involves replacement of this collagen with improved optical function. Overuse of topical steroid can inhibit collagen synthesis and impair healing.

Endothelial cells are terminally differentiated and do not replicate. Repair is by enlargement of existing cells and migration to fill an area of cell loss. This results in reduced cell density, larger cells and variation in shape (polymegathism).

1.2.4 Conjunctiva

1.2.4.1 Regions

The superior and inferior conjunctiva consist of three different regions: palpebral, fornix and bulbar. The normal conjunctival sac is deeper superiorly (14 mm) than inferiorly (11 mm).

1.2.4.2 Layers

The conjunctiva consists of an epithelial and a stromal layer (Fig. 1.2). The epithelium is formed by two to four layers of stratified cells resting on a basement membrane. Immediately peripheral to the limbus superiorly and inferiorly are the palisades of Vogt, which are thought to be the primary location of stem cells contributing epithelial cells to the cornea. Mucin-secreting goblet cells are found within the deeper epithelial layer mainly of the fornix and palpebral conjunctiva. The conjunctival stroma lies beneath the epithelium and consists of a highly vascularised adenoid layer containing mast cells and other inflammatory cells and a deep fibrous layer harbouring larger blood vessels and nerves. In the palpebral conjunctiva the fibrous layer is replaced by the tarsal plates.

1.2.4.3 Immunology

The conjunctiva is a highly immunologically active tissue that can mount a range of reactions in response to infection, allergy and inflammation. These reactions are characterised by structural changes, including the formation of papillae (hypertrophy with central blood vessel) and follicle formation (clusters of lymphocytes and macrophages).

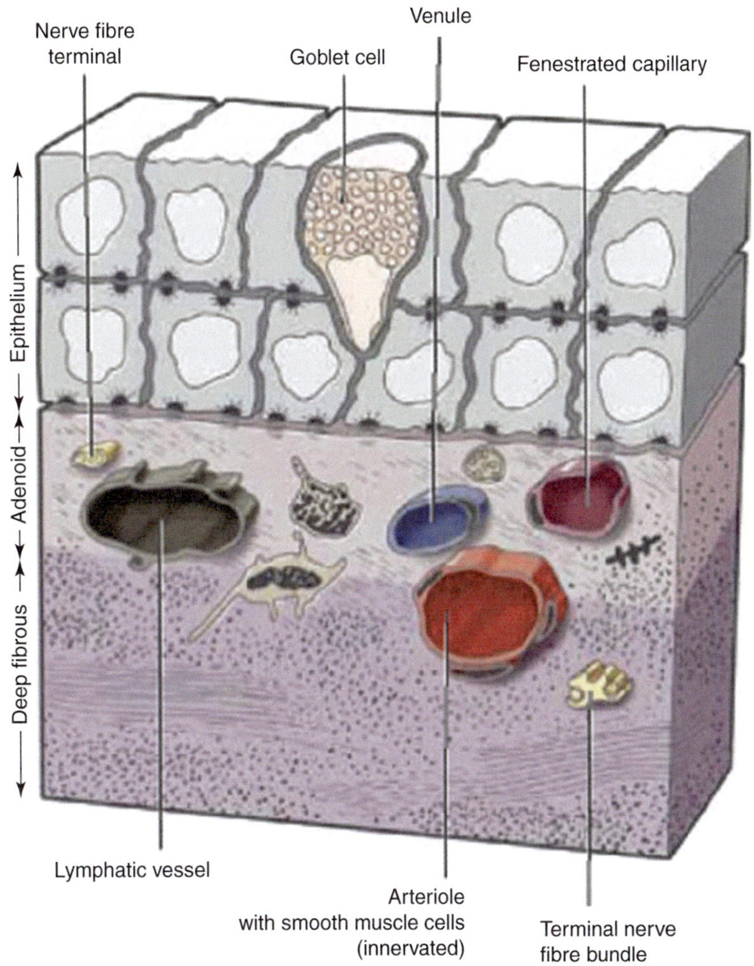

Fig. 1.2 Illustration of conjunctival anatomy

1.2.4.4 Circulation

The blood supply of the conjunctiva is from the palpebral branches of the dorso-nasal and lacrimal arteries (palpebral region) and the anterior ciliary arteries (bulbar region). In anterior uveitis or severe keratitis, the deep ciliary vessels are engorged. The conjunctiva is richly supplied with lymphatics, with a temporal direction of lymph flow, and a venous drainage system through a number of routes including the anterior ciliary veins, the inferior ophthalmic vein and a superior and post-tarsal venous plexus.

1.2.4.5 Innervation

The sensory innervation of the conjunctiva is through touch-sensitive corpuscles mainly located in the limbal conjunctival epithelium and autonomic innervation with sympathetic and parasympathetic terminals in the walls of arterioles and capillaries.

1.3 Anaesthesia for Corneal Surgery

1.3.1 Topical Anaesthesia

Topical anaesthesia is suitable for minor surgery on an otherwise healthy eye. This includes excimer laser procedures, removal of corneal sutures or foreign bodies. Available drugs include (in order of increasing anaesthetic potency) proxymetacaine, lignocaine, oxybuprocaine, tetracaine (amethocaine) (Table 1.2). These

Table 1.2 Topical anaesthetics

	Potency	Approximate duration (min)	Discomfort
Proxymetacaine (0.5 %)	Mild	15	Minor
Lignocaine (4 %)	Moderate	20	Mild
Oxybuprocaine (0.4 %)	Strong	30	Significant
Tetracaine (1 %)	Strong	30	Moderate

Table 1.3 Local blocks and general anaesthesia

Type	Advantages	Disadvantages
Sub-Tenon	Safe, low rate of complications, good anaesthesia	Sub-conjunctival haemorrhage, chemosis, asymmetric akinesia with globe displacement. May be difficult in the presence of an encircling band from a previous retinal detachment repair. Care required if the sclera is thin in pathological myopia
Peribulbar	Avoids sub-conjunctival haemorrhage and chemosis. Good akinesia	Raised intraorbital and intraocular pressure. Risk of retrobulbar haemorrhage (treat with lateral cantholysis). Risk of globe perforation. Risk of intravascular injection. Risk of intradural anaesthetic and brainstem anaesthesia if inadvertently given into the optic nerve dural sheath (especially with retrobulbar block; complication managed by anaesthetist as requires intubation and circulatory support until wears off; blocks should therefore be performed predominantly by anaesthetist or with anaesthetist present)
General	Excellent control of operative conditions; avoids the risks associated with local blocks; usually well tolerated and quick to wear off	Increased risk of cardiorespiratory morbidity, especially in elderly patients; minor trauma to lips or teeth; greater need for personnel (anaesthetist, anaesthetic assistant/technician) and equipment; greater time requirement for induction of and recovery from anaesthesia; may require overnight stay rather than day-case surgery. Coughing/vomiting postoperatively may raise intraocular pressure or displace DSEK graft

agents also interrupt tight junctions between epithelial cells and render the epithelium more permeable to water, which may result in transient mild haze. They also make the epithelium more permeable to other drugs and enhance their absorption into the anterior chamber, for example, antibiotics. One or two drops are instilled into the lower fornix, and the onset of action for all is rapid (within seconds).

1.3.2 Local Block

Sub-Tenon and peribulbar anaesthesia both give more profound and prolonged anaesthesia than topical agents with various degrees of akinesia (Table 1.3). Sub-Tenon injections are more effective at achieving anaesthesia as the drug is delivered close to the ciliary nerves, so a smaller volume can be given, but often there is only moderate akinesia. Peribulbar block is more effective at achieving akinesia as the anaesthetic has better access to the third, fourth and sixth cranial nerves which control the extra-ocular motility. Both types of injection require patient's cooperation and therefore are less suitable for children or adults who cannot be relied upon to remain still throughout the procedure.

1.3.2.1 Sub-Tenon's Block

With the patient supine topical anaesthetic is given and a lid speculum placed. The patient is directed to elevate and abduct the eye. The conjunctiva and Tenons are grasped with a Moorfields forceps 5 mm from the infero-nasal limbus and snipped with Westcott scissors to open a pocket into the sub-Tenon's space. Blunt dissection with Westcott scissors is used to extend this space posteriorly. A curved blunt 'sub-Tenon's cannula' (Fig. 1.3) is advanced posteriorly into this space until the syringe and cannula are vertical, and the anaesthetic is injected slowly. There should be no reflux and no chemosis as this may indicate sub-conjunctival administration.

1.3.2.2 Peribulbar Block

With the patient supine, topical anaesthesia is given. The classical site for injection is located at the junction of the medial 2/3 and lateral 1/3 of the inferior orbital margin, just inside the bony orbital rim (Fig. 1.4). This ensures that the sharp needle will be directed into the orbit where the distance between the globe and bone is greatest for safety. An alternative route is medial to the caruncle. The 25 mm 25G needle is oriented vertically and advanced into the orbit either through the lid skin or through the conjunctiva of the lower fornix until the tip is beyond the equator of the globe. The patient is directed to move the eye to show it has not been touched by the needle. Four to five millilitres of anaesthetic is given (very slowly since a sudden rise in intraorbital pressure is very uncomfortable) and the needle withdrawn. There should be no firm resistance to insertion of the needle or administration of the anaesthetic; if this is encountered, globe perforation should be suspected and excluded with indirect ophthalmoscopy.

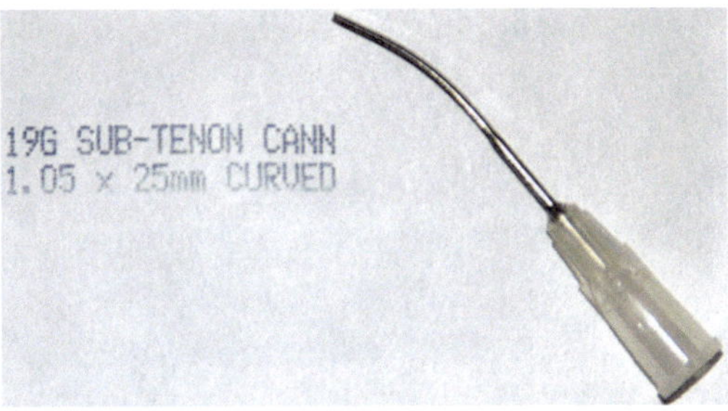

Fig. 1.3 Sub-Tenon's cannula

Depending on the duration of anaesthesia required, lignocaine (shorter duration) or a 50:50 mixture of lignocaine and levobupivacaine (longer duration) can be given. Lignocaine is safer as the therapeutic window is wider. Some practitioners advocate the addition of hyalase (150–300 units) to the anaesthetic to aid diffusion throughout orbital tissue, although this results in longer postoperative diplopia. Pre-warming of the anaesthetic to body temperature reduces discomfort and gives faster onset of effect.

A Honan balloon (30 mmHg) can be used after sub-Tenon or peribulbar technique to encourage diffusion of anaesthetic and minimise the rise in IOP. The indication to use a Honan balloon should be restricted in the presence of arterial disease or glaucoma.

Comments

1. Sharp needle techniques should avoid the superior orbit to avoid traumatising vascular structures.
2. Avoid both sub-Tenon's and peribulbar blocks when anaesthetising the eye for repair of ruptured globe or corneal perforation as raised intraorbital and intraocular pressure may expel globe contents. Always prepare intravenous access in these cases.

1.3.3 General Anaesthesia

All general anaesthetics reduce intraocular pressure, which may aid surgery. General anaesthesia may be combined with neuromuscular blockade, but this is not essential. Relative indications for GA include 'open globe' procedures, particularly

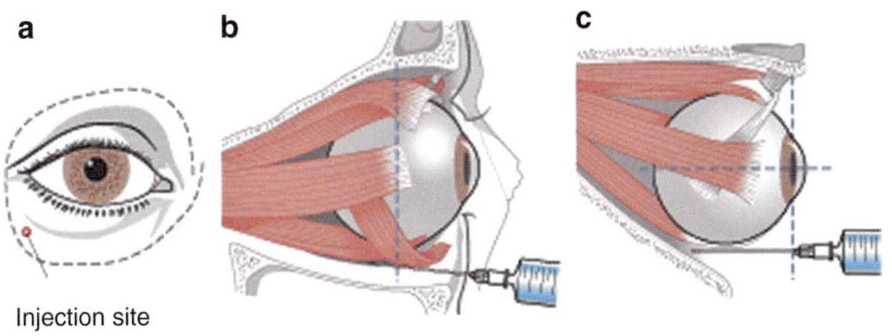

Fig. 1.4 Peribulbar block. (**a**) Injection site; (**b**) Lateral view; (**c**) Medial view

repair of trauma and PKP; inability to comply with local anaesthetic; refusal of local anaesthesia; marked head tremor; inability to lie still for sufficient time; and long or potentially uncomfortable procedures.

1.4 Suturing

1.4.1 Needles

Needles for corneal sutures come in a range of profiles. Spatulated needles separate laminae of tissue parallel to the passage of the needle. These needles are suitable for repairing corneal lacerations. Round bodied needles leave a small suture track and are suitable for conjunctival suturing. Needles come in ½ circle or 3/8 circle and usually have a circular shape. A small radius of curvature helps pass short, deep bites, whereas a larger radius of curvature results in longer bites more suitable for sutures in the peripheral cornea.

1.4.2 Suture Material

The three most commonly used suture materials in corneal surgery include nylon, polyglycolic acid and polyester (Table 1.4).

Table 1.4 Suture material

Material	Characteristics	Typical indication
Nylon	Nylon is non-absorbable and mostly used in size 10/0 or 11/0. Finer sutures, such as 11/0, alter topography less but are more likely to break. Nylon is hydrolysed slowly and thins over a period of 12–24 months	Penetrating keratoplasty Corneal laceration
Polyglycolic acid (Vicryl®)	Vicryl® sutures are absorbable, lose tensile strength after about 7–10 days and are completely absorbed within 2–3 months. The fine size 10/0 is harder to handle than 10/0 nylon, as it retains memory of shape and tends to coil. However, it is suitable when required for short duration, for example, for phacoemulsification wounds or to secure an amniotic membrane	Leaking corneal wound after phacoemul sification
Polyester (Mersilene®)	Mersilene® is a non-absorbable suture made from braided polyester and available in 10/0 and 11/0 on spatulated needles	

1.4.3 General Principles

The needle is grasped by the tips of the needle holders in the middle of the curve of the needle's body. The needle tip enters perpendicular to the epithelial surface and is guided through the stroma along a tract determined by the shape of the needle. This should result in minimal distortion of tissue. The suture tract should pass through 95 % stromal depth (Fig. 1.5). Full-thickness sutures must be avoided as this creates a pathway along which microbes can enter the anterior chamber and cause endophthalmitis. Entry and exit points should be equidistant either side of the base of the wound to ensure endothelial apposition. Spacing between adjacent sutures should be slightly less than the length of the bite. After securing with a non-slip knot, the ends should be trimmed short and the suture rotated so that the knot is buried within the stroma.

1.4.4 Interrupted Sutures

The suture is placed to lie perpendicular to the wound. Entry and exit should be at least 1 mm from the wound edge (Fig. 1.6). Adjacent sutures

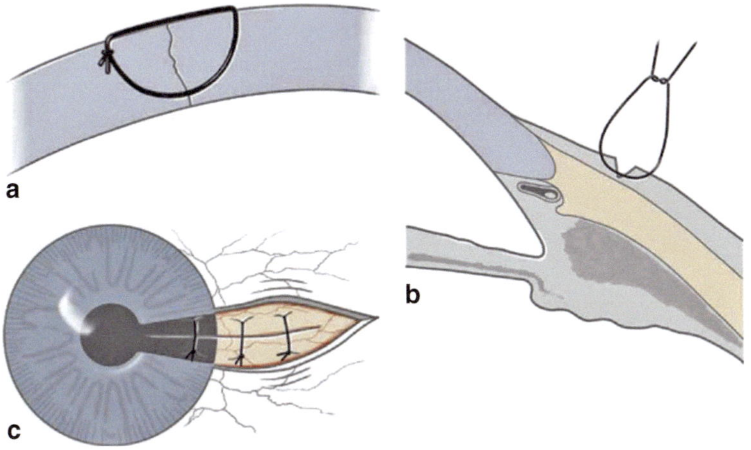

Fig. 1.5 Illustration of corneal, conjunctival and scleral suture techniques for lacerations. (**a**) Corneal suture; (**b**) Conjunctival suture; (**c**) Scleral suture

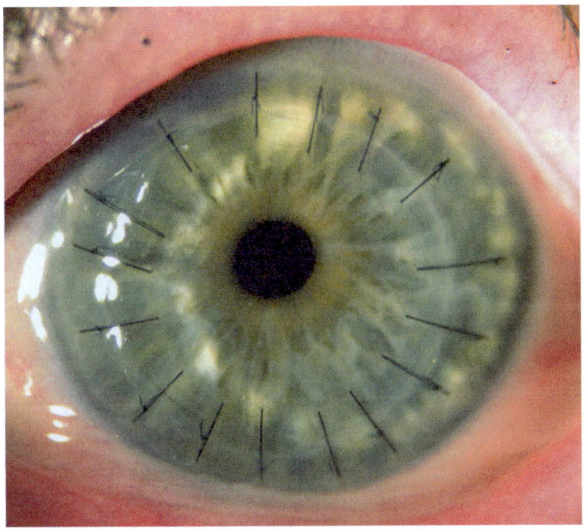

Fig. 1.6 Interrupted sutures for PKP for Fuchs endothelial dystrophy

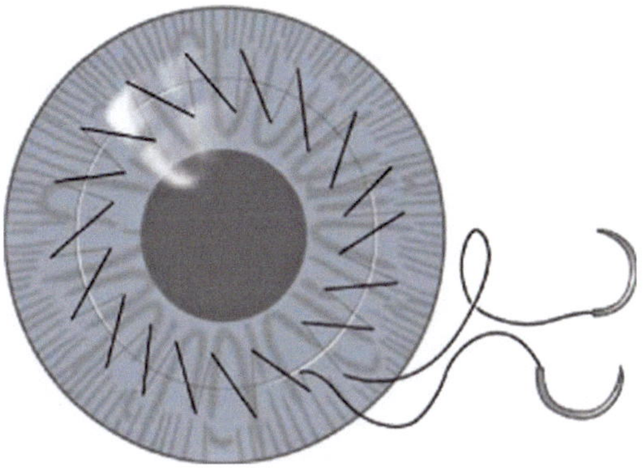

Fig. 1.7 Illustration of penetrating keratoplasty: start and end of running suture

are placed just less than a bite-length apart to ensure no gaps between the 'compression zones' of adjacent sutures.

This technique is easier to learn and has the advantage of allowing sutures to be removed individually to adjust astigmatism, if there is vascularisation or infiltrate affecting a suture tract or if a suture comes loose or breaks. However, it is slower and may result in irregular astigmatism due to uneven tension along a long corneal wound. However, postoperative corneal astigmatism, as measured with topography, can be reduced with adding interrupted sutures to the flatter meridian (as a second procedure) or removing individual sutures from the steeper meridian.

1.4.5 Continuous Sutures

Continuous (running) sutures are used to secure corneal grafts, such as PKP, DALK and tectonic grafts. Bites are again oriented perpendicular to the wound edges (Fig. 1.7). Typically 16 bites are placed around the circumference of a 7.5 mm corneal graft to give appropriate spacing (Fig. 1.8); sometimes more bites are placed (Fig. 1.9). Parts of the suture must be rotated once completed to bury the knot in the donor cornea.

The continuous suture technique is quicker (e.g. for PKP) but is technically harder, and the surgeon must ensure that the needle tip is not touched by the forceps as this will blunt it and make suture bites towards the end harder to place, requiring more force and potentially bending the

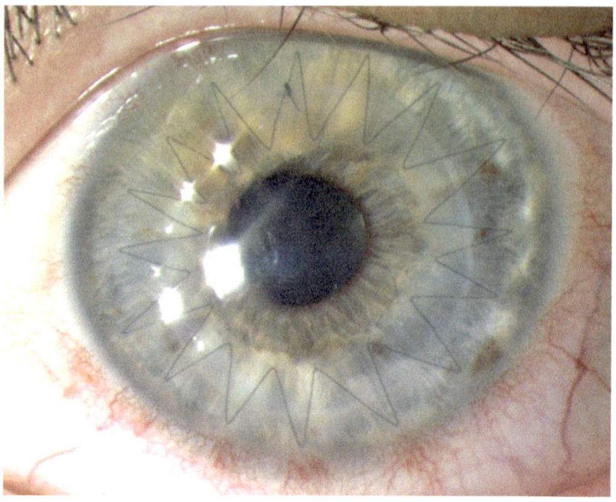

Fig. 1.8 16 bit running suture 1 week postoperative

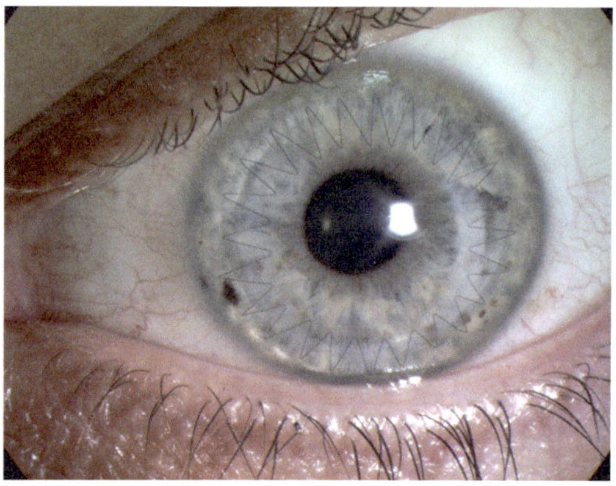

Fig. 1.9 24 bit running suture 12 months postoperative

needle. Tension can be distributed to minimise astigmatism and may be adjusted later according to on-table or postoperative topography. Care must be taken however not to pull across the edge of the forceps or apply too much force to the suture to prevent breakage. Loosening of the suture may be countered by placing a separate, intrastromal 'loop tensioning' 10/0 nylon suture to re-tension the continuous suture.

When indicated, removal of a continuous suture is easier than removal of many interrupted sutures. If the suture breaks, becomes too superficial (Fig. 1.10) or suture tract infiltration is seen (Fig. 1.11) before the suture is due to be removed, it may be necessary to return the patient to the operating theatre for removal and re-suturing (usually with interrupted sutures).

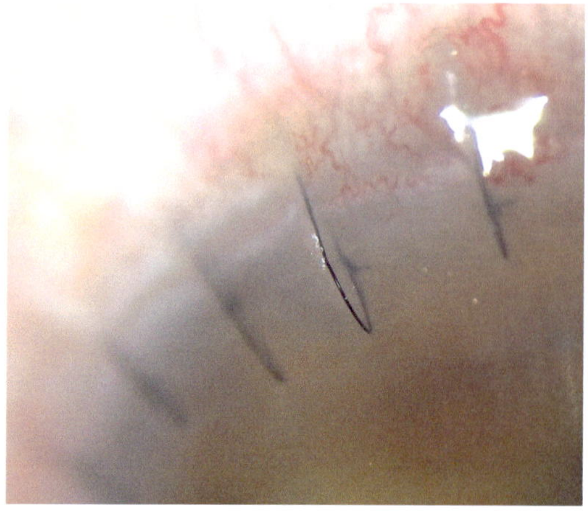

Fig. 1.10 Loose interrupted suture

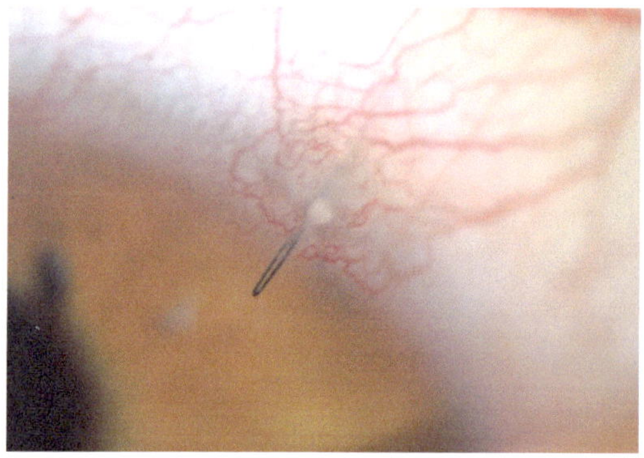

Fig. 1.11 Suture infiltrate

A single continuous suture may exert a torque on the graft if the sutures are placed radially; for this reason double continuous sutures running in opposite directions may be combined to eliminate this. The obvious disadvantages of this are the extra time involved and the increased number of suture passes through the stroma with the risk of the second needle cutting a suture already in place.

1.4.6 Suture Adjustment

The tension in a corneal suture will influence the corneal refractive power in its meridian. A tight suture will steepen the corneal curvature and increase the refractive power, whereas a loose suture will have the opposite effect. This can be used to modify corneal astigmatism. The effect of a given suture will be more marked the closer it is to the visual axis. Selective removal of interrupted sutures can be used to correct an excessively steep corneal axis. With a continuous suture, the bites in the steep meridian can be loosened by rotating the suture from the flat meridian, which is in turn tightened. Suture adjustment should be performed as early as is practical (ideally within 2 weeks) before wound healing is complete so that the change in tension can influence subsequent collagen remodelling. This is done under topical anaesthesia and is best done under the operating microscope so that on-table keratoscopy can be used to judge the end point. Suture adjustment breaks the epithelium so topical antibiotic cover must be given after the procedure. The effect can be assessed by serial topography examinations and repeated as necessary.

1.4.7 Suture Removal

Corneal sutures can be removed under topical anaesthesia at the slit lamp or under the operating microscope. The latter may offer greater comfort for both surgeon and patient if there are many remaining sutures or a continuous suture or if the procedure is likely to be of long duration. It is also more convenient if the patient is susceptible to vasovagal episodes or cannot be relied upon to remain sufficiently still at the slit lamp (e.g. elderly, mild head tremor, anxious patient squeezing strongly).

Topical anaesthesia is applied and the superficial pass of a suture is cut (on the host side) with a 21G needle or fine blade. There is necessarily disturbance of the epithelium to achieve this as the epithelium heals over the suture. One free end is grasped in a fine non-toothed forceps and the suture removed so as to draw the knot out through the stroma on the same side of the wound on which it lies. This avoids attempting to draw the knot through the stromal scar, which may cause dehiscence. Exceptions to this are cases where there is suspected suture tract infection, in which case the direction of removal should be such that potentially infected material is drawn away from, rather than through, donor cornea. A firm, sharp tug is more effective at removing the suture cleanly than steady gentle traction.

Interrupted sutures can be removed selectively to reduce astigmatism (see above) during the remodelling phase. Once healing is complete both interrupted and continuous sutures should be removed. In rare cases where wound healing is very slow or the integrity of the interface is in doubt (for instance patients taking systemic steroids or the very elderly), sutures can be left in situ indefinitely.

Loose sutures should be removed as they will trap mucus leading to vascularisation and increased risk of infection or corneal graft rejection. A loose suture does not contribute to wound stability, and hence its removal will not compromise wound integrity. Vascularisation of or infiltrate invading of a suture tract should also prompt removal of the suture. Broken sutures must also be removed once identified as the protruding end(s) will cause discomfort.

The main complications of suture removal are listed in Table 1.5.

1.4.8 Sutureless Surgery

Small corneal incisions can be created so that they self-seal without the need for sutures. This relies on surgical technique in the construction of the wound, adequate intraocular pressure to assist wound apposition and patient cooperation not to rub the eye while the incision is healing. This is most frequently seen in phacoemulsification surgery but also contributes to wound stability in DSEK.

1.5 Corneal Examination

1.5.1 Slit-Lamp Examination

Slit-lamp examination should begin at low magnification to obtain an overview of the eyelid margins, fornices and anterior segment. Higher magnification can then be used for more detailed examination (Table 1.6).

Table 1.5 Complications of suture removal

Complication	Management
Wound dehiscence	Wound dehiscence requires prompt re-suturing. A small dehiscence may be re-sutured under local anaesthesia, but a more significant defect may require general anaesthesia to prevent prolapse of ocular tissues. If the anterior chamber has collapsed, it should be reformed with viscoelastic which is removed at the end of the procedure. Inadequate wound healing may allow slippage of the wound edges when sutures are removed. If this creates a symptomatic step, re-suturing should be undertaken
Retained suture material	Suture material may be retained if the knot comes loose as it is drawn through the cornea or if the suture breaks under tension. Attempts should be made to ensure that any remaining material is sufficiently clear of the surface to avoid foreign body discomfort resulting from a protruding end. Retained suture material is unlikely to cause significant adverse reactions as nylon is biologically inert
Infection	Infection may develop after suture removal since the epithelium will be breached. Prophylactic broad-spectrum topical antibiotic should be applied after all suture removal procedures until the epithelium heals. In cases where the suture tract is already infected or there are signs of infection, intensive broad-spectrum topical antibiotic should be given for 1 week following suture removal. Infection in a corneal graft greatly increases the risk of rejection so topical steroid may be necessary
Change in refraction	The change in tension in the wound once sutures are removed may result in a change in refraction, particularly astigmatism. This may be uneven depending on how uniform healing has been within the wound. The patient should be warned of this and advised against obtaining new spectacles until the refraction has stabilised. Further interventions may also be planned once the refraction has stabilised

Table 1.6 Anterior segment examination

Structure	Signs
Lids	Entropion/ectropion. Notch. Blepharitis. Sub-tarsal foreign body. Laxity/floppy eyelid syndrome
Lashes	Trichiasis, distichiasis
Puncta	Presence, patency, position. Plug present
Fornices	Symblepharon, fornix shortening. Giant fornix syndrome
Tarsal conjunctiva	Follicles, papillae, injection
Bulbar conjunctiva	Injection, pterygium, tumour, scars, cysts
Sclera	Inflammation, thinning/melt
Limbus	Limbitis, limbal ischaemia, pannus
Corneal nerves	Perineural infiltrates
Tear film	Quality, BUT, dellen, debris
Epithelium	Microcysts, filaments, dystrophy, foreign body, oedema, abrasion, ulcer, band keratopathy, punctate erosions, inflammation
Stroma	Dystrophy, scar, thickness, oedema, infiltrate, ulcer, abscess, neovascularisation
Descemet's membrane	Dystrophy, scar, striae
Endothelium	Cell morphology (specular reflection), dystrophy, endotheliitis

BUT break-up time

The illumination can be used in different ways:

- Diffuse illumination gives a good overview of the anterior segment structures. Low magnification and a wide beam are used. Avoid excessive illumination as this will be uncomfortable for the patient.
- Direct illumination with a wide beam is used to examine the surface, a narrower beam for assessing a section. The depth of a corneal lesion can also be determined. Start with low magnification and increase if necessary. The measuring scale can be used to measure a lesion (e.g. the size of an ulcer), but the beam and microscope must be coaxial and directed from the 'straight-ahead' position to be accurate.
- Indirect illumination is useful for assessing corneal nerves, subtle opacities and dystrophies.
- Retro-illumination (from the retina or iris) is useful for examining corneal dystrophies located at the epithelial basement membrane or the Descemet's layer.
- Sclerotic scatter: The observation and illumination systems are uncoupled and the beam

Table 1.7 Schirmer test

Tear production	Distance of wetting (mm)
Low	<5
Moderate	5–10
Normal	>10

directed at the limbus while the observer views the apex of the cornea. This shows areas of subtle oedema or opacity.
- Specular reflection: The observation and illumination systems are positioned at equal angular displacement either side of the midline. The endothelium can be examined if the magnification is increased and viewing is monocular.

1.5.2 Schirmer Test

This test assesses the quantity of tear secretion (basal and reflex) and is hence a useful test for aqueous deficiency. It is used in the diagnosis of dry eye and is part of the standard preoperative assessment for patients requesting laser refractive surgery. To assess combined basal and reflex tearing, a standard filter paper strip with preprinted scale is placed in the inferior fornix and the patient instructed to blink normally but not to dab the eye. The paper is removed after 5 min and the distance of wetting measured (Table 1.7). To assess basal tear production, topical anaesthetic is instilled before placement of the paper strip.

1.5.3 Tear Break-Up Time

Measurement of tear break-up time is indicated in the work-up of patients with symptoms of dry eye and provides information regarding the stability of the tear film. The patient is examined at the slit lamp under high magnification, and fluorescein is used to stain the tear film. The patient is instructed to take one normal blink and then not to blink. The time taken for localised dry spots to appear in the tear film is recorded (Table 1.8). An unstable tear film may be due to mucin deficiency or abnormalities of the lipid layer allowing rapid tear evaporation.

Table 1.8 Tear break-up time

Tear film stability	Break-up time (s)
Low	<5
Moderate	5–15
Normal	>15

1.5.4 Corneal Sensitivity

Assessment of corneal sensitivity is useful in the assessment of dry eyes and other conditions potentially affecting corneal sensitivity including herpetic keratitis, diabetes and disorders of the trigeminal nerve. In its simplest form, it consists of observing whether the patient can feel a wisp of a cotton bud touching the cornea. A quantitative test may be carried out with the Cochet-Bonnet aesthesiometer which relies on the deformation of a 0.12 mm thick nylon filament of variable length (0–60 mm) in contact with the cornea to provide a standardised touch stimulus. Stimulating pressures range between 973 and 17,699 mg/mm^2. The shorter the filament required for the patient to perceive the touch, the less sensitive the cornea.

Reduced corneal sensitivity is a risk factor for both compromise of the epithelium's barrier function and breakdown of the epithelium itself. This predisposes the patient to microbial keratitis, stromal melt and corneal perforation. If loss of corneal sensation is identified, the patient must be advised to use regular lubricants to maintain an optimal environment for the compromised ocular surface.

1.5.5 Pachymetry

Pachymetry is the measurement of the corneal thickness and has a number of applications:
- In the correction of intraocular pressure recorded by applanation tonometry. Topical steroids are used frequently after corneal surgery and can induce rises in intraocular pressure; accurate monitoring is essential to avoid glaucomatous visual loss.
- In the assessment for suitability for LASIK. Patients with thin corneas are at risk of

postoperative ectasia and should be counselled towards surface treatments (LASEK).

- To assess for corneal oedema in cases of suspected graft rejection or endothelial dysfunction.

There are several techniques to determine the corneal thickness:

Ultrasound: A beam of ultrasound (20 MHz) is delivered at the cornea by a contact probe. The time between transmission of a pulse and detection of its reflection from the posterior corneal surface is measured, and since the speed of sound through corneal tissue is known, the distance travelled can be calculated. The ultrasound probe can be placed at any part of the cornea but is best used for the central corneal thickness measurement. A number of readings are taken in quick succession and a mean is calculated. The technique is fast and easy and is relatively user independent.

Oculus Pentacam: This is a noncontact method of imaging the anterior segment which uses a rotating Scheimpflug camera to construct a 3D image of the anterior segment. Multiple slit images are taken which are integrated by a computer. Software is able to produce corneal pachymetry maps as well as topography data.

Bausch and Lomb Orbscan: This system uses a scanning slit technique to obtain images of the anterior and posterior corneal surfaces. Placido rings are projected onto the cornea, and the reflected images are detected as the slit beams move across the cornea. In addition to pachymetry measurements, data are produced about the corneal topography and refractive power of 3, 5 and 7 mm optical zones. This takes longer and is more user dependent than ultrasound but gives a pachymetry map of the whole cornea. Orbscan tends to under-read compared to ultrasound so this may be preferred when considering suitability for excimer laser procedures.

Optical Coherence Tomography (OCT): OCT is based on the principle of interference between one light beam reflected from ocular structures (index beam) and one travelling along a reference path. The difference in phase between the two signals received by the detector allows the distance travelled by the index beam to be calculated. An image is built up from thousands of data points and displayed as a 'slice' through the eye. The signals from anterior and posterior corneal surfaces allow the creation of a pachymetry map which shows corneal thickness across the whole cornea.

There is variation in recorded thicknesses between different modalities so care must be exercised when comparing measurements over time. It is more reliable to take serial measurements with the same device.

1.5.6 Keratometry

Keratometry is the measurement of the radius of curvature (r) of the anterior corneal surface, from which the refractive power (D) can be estimated using the following equation with the refractive indexes of the cornea (n_2; clinically adopted 'average' of 1.3755) and air (n_1):

$$D = \frac{n_2 - n_1}{r} = \frac{1.3375 - 1}{r}$$

1.5.6.1 Javal Keratometer

Keratometers use the anterior corneal surface as a powerful convex mirror. The Javal-Schiotz keratometer has been the most widely used keratometer for many years, but newer automated devices are now available. Illuminated mires are projected onto the cornea, and their first Purkinje images are aligned in the two axes. The images are doubled to compensate for small eye movements. Once the images are aligned, the radius of curvature and corneal power can be read off the scales. Correct alignment of the mires will also allow the axis of astigmatism to be measured. This only assesses the central 3 mm optical zone. For assessment of corneal shapes in the periphery, topography is more appropriate.

1.5.6.2 Handheld Keratometer

For example, the Nidek KM-500 is a small, handheld and automatic keratometer providing quick readings (Fig. 1.12). Because of its design, it is very useful for wheelchair patients or lying patients (e.g. during an operation). The data can be transmitted via infrared to a printer.

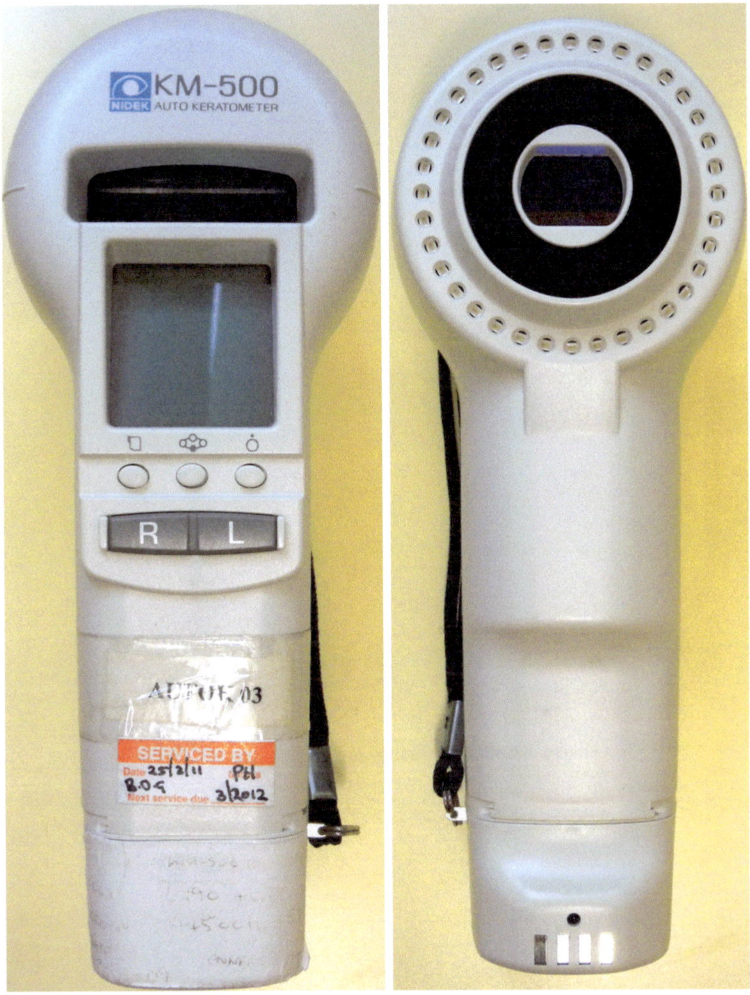

Fig. 1.12 Photo of handheld keratometer Nidek KM-500

1.5.7 Corneal Topography (Placido Ring Based)

Topography is the assessment of the shape of the corneal surface. Measurement systems may be based on assessment of point height or surface slope. Placido-ring-based systems (e.g. Zeiss Atlas: Fig. 1.13; Topcon CA-200: Fig. 1.14; and Topcon KR8100P: Fig. 1.15) project a pattern, usually multiple series of points or concentric rings of light, onto the cornea and analyse the reflected images. Where the lines of the reflected image are closer together, the steepness of curvature of the cornea is greater. The output is in the form of colour-coded 'contour' maps analogous to contour lines on a geographical map, but indicating curvature at a given point rather than elevation (Fig. 1.16). The output may also include numerical assessment of corneal astigmatism (simulated Ks) and the axes of astigmatism. Comparison of results to a normative database allows qualitative assessment of overall corneal morphology and can alert the clinician to particular conditions, for example, keratoconus. However, no assessment can be made of the posterior corneal surface or corneal thickness.

1.5.7.1 Bausch and Lomb Orbscan

The Orbscan (Fig. 1.17) uses two types of measurements: a Placido-ring-based system (as above) and a scanning slit beam which records data from both anterior and posterior corneal surfaces, enabling a pachymetry map to be generated.

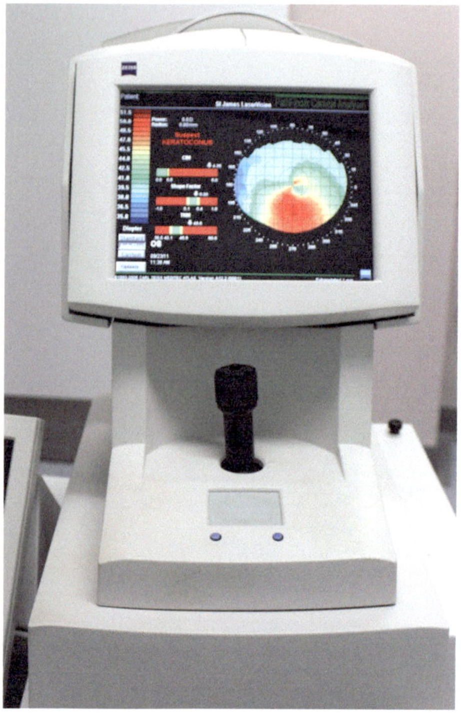

Fig. 1.13 Zeiss Atlas corneal topographer

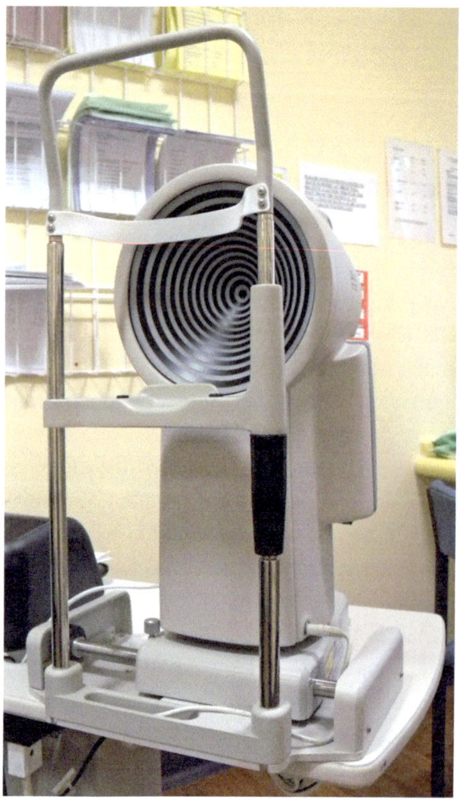

Fig. 1.14 Topcon CA-200 corneal topographer

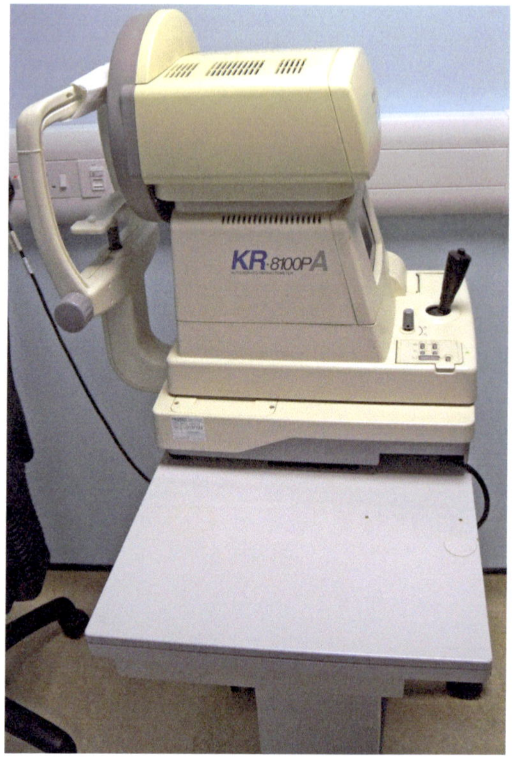

Fig. 1.15 Topcon KR 8100P corneal topographer

Analysis of the data points is in terms of elevation from a reference plane which allows greater accuracy in identifying small variations. The slope and curvature at a given point can then be extrapolated from the raw data. The usual reference plane is a best-fit sphere, and each point is compared to this to determine whether it falls above, on or below the reference. Again, colour-coded maps are produced as a graphical display of data to facilitate analysis. The output can be customised according to user preference; the usual dataset would show anterior and posterior 'float' (i.e. deviation from the reference plane for anterior and posterior corneal surfaces, respectively), curvature and pachymetry (Fig. 1.18). Its advantages include imaging of the posterior surface which may enable early detection of keratoconus (posterior elevation > 40 μm), and it is able to image a large area of the corneal surface. The main disadvantage of the scanning slit is that the images are separated from each other, that is, there is no common reference point. Image capture also takes longer than

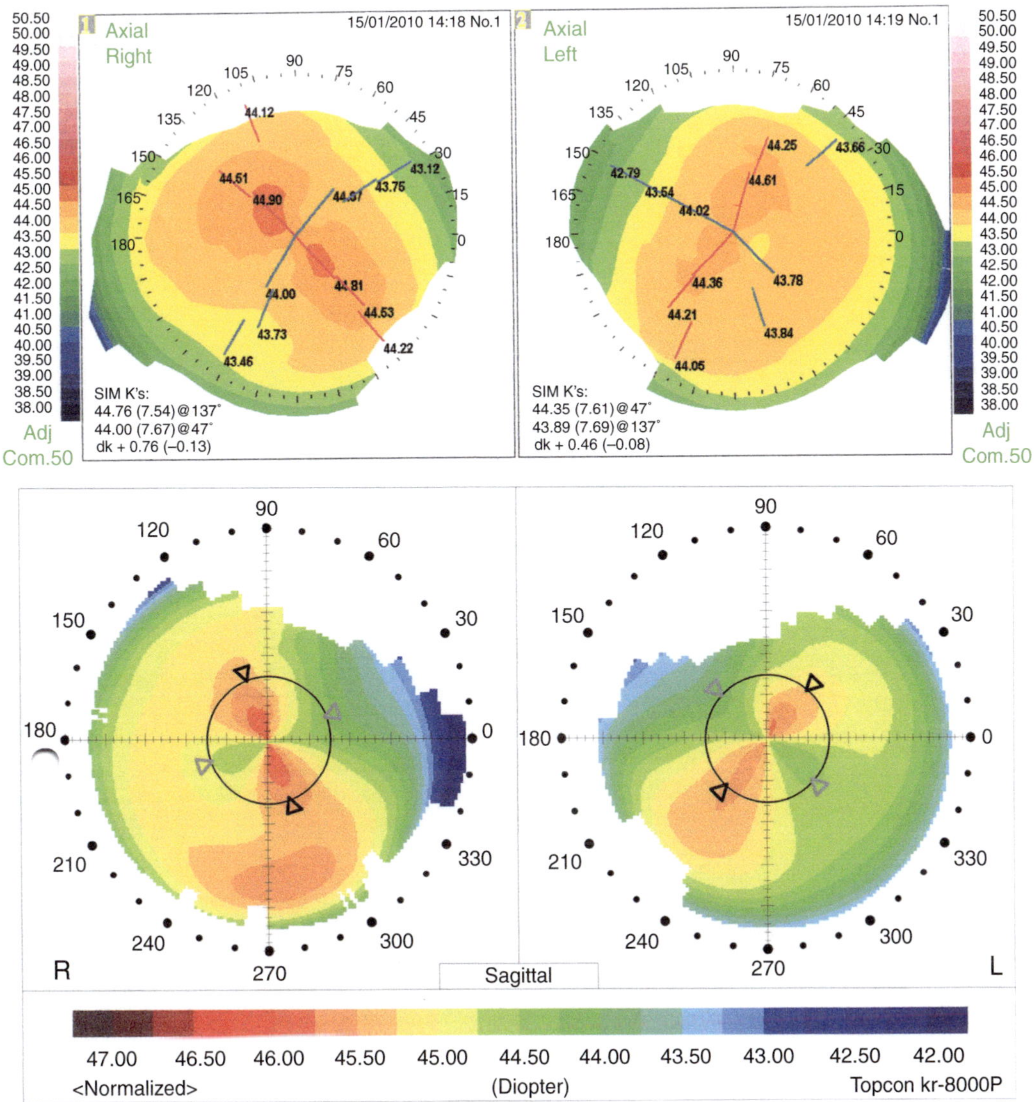

Fig. 1.16 Printouts from Nidek OPD scan (*top*) and Topcon KR-8000P (*bottom*)

Placido-ring-based imaging or video-keratoscopy, so it may not be suitable for very young or elderly patients or those with tremor or poor fixation.

1.5.7.2 Topcon CA-200

This is a stand-alone topographer using a Placido-ring system. The device is controlled by a touch screen that makes acquisition, operation and evaluation of the cornea fast and easy (Fig. 1.14).

1.5.8 Corneal Topography (Scheimpflug)

Scheimpflug imaging is a contact-free technique for obtaining clear images when the object plane, lens plane and image plane are not parallel. The camera system rotates around a fixed central point and uses a scanning slit to capture multiple optical slice images. In this case though, the images all have a common reference point and are therefore

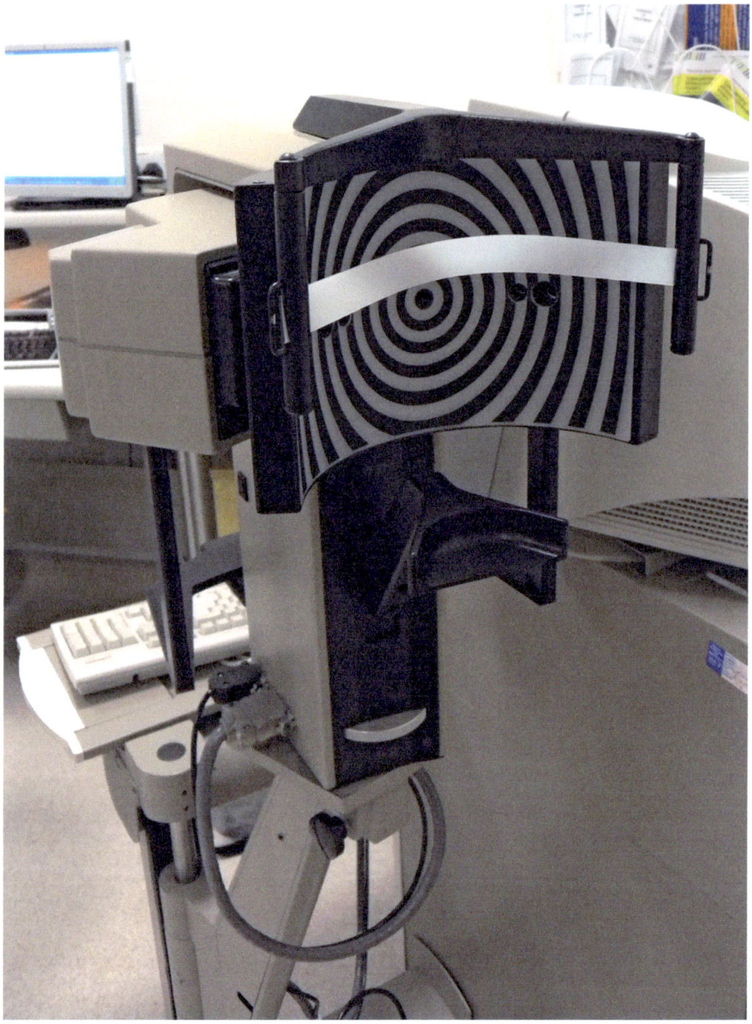

Fig. 1.17 Bausch and Lomb Orbscan corneal topographer

linked which gives greater accuracy in detailed data analysis and graphical representation. Data are again captured for anterior and posterior corneal surface maps (enabling pachymetry mapping), but the resolution is higher than that of the Orbscan. The Scheimpflug systems currently available also image the iridocorneal angle and the anterior and posterior chamber, allowing observation as far as the posterior lens surface.

1.5.8.1 Oculus Pentacam

The Pentacam system (Figs. 1.19 and 1.20) was one of the first on the market and has become a reference for Scheimpflug-based topography. Different models and software packages are available: cataract package, refractive package, contact lens fitting and 3D pIOL simulation. The resolution of the Pentacam HR is five times that of the other Pentacam models, and it offers quicker image acquisition (<2 s for a complete scan). The results can be visualised in many different ways (Figs. 1.21, 1.22 and 1.23).

1.5.8.2 Ziemer Galilei and Schwind Sirius

The Galilei and Sirius systems combine (dual and single) Scheimpflug cameras with a Placido-ring-based projection system for higher accuracy in relation to elevation and curvature data (Fig. 1.24). The dual cameras compensate for eye movement during acquisition and reduce any measurement errors incurred when the projected slit is decentred away from the corneal

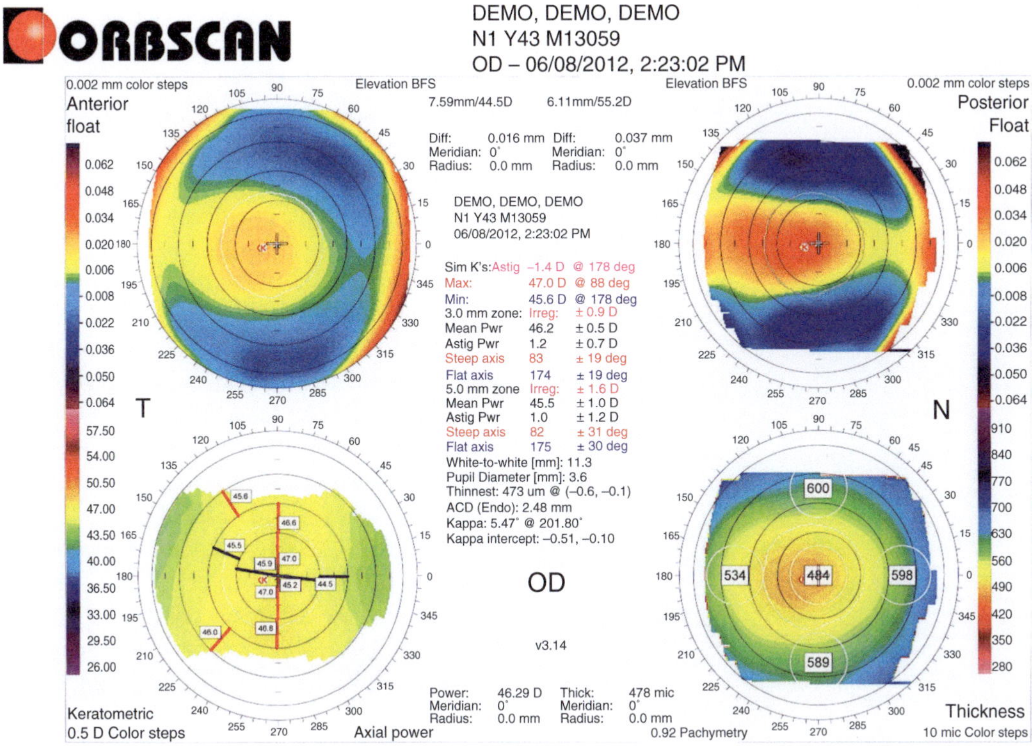

Fig. 1.18 Printout from Orbscan

vertex. By merging the datasets from the Scheimpflug cameras and from the Placido detection, a single dataset is generated which gives greater accuracy in assessing elevation and curvature readings. An integral near/far target allows imaging of the relaxed eye and the accommodating eye for comparison. The Schwind system also enables measurements of pupil diameters at different light conditions.

Graphical output can be presented as colour-coded topography/pachymetry maps (Fig. 1.25) or as a 3D reconstruction of the ocular structure in question. The mentioned devices are noncontact methods but are user dependent and do require a degree of cooperation and the ability to fixate by the patient. Images and data may be useful in diagnosis or in monitoring progression over time.

1.5.9 Aberrometry

The measurements of irregularities in the eye's refracting system are termed aberrometry. Aberrations range from spherical and cylindrical

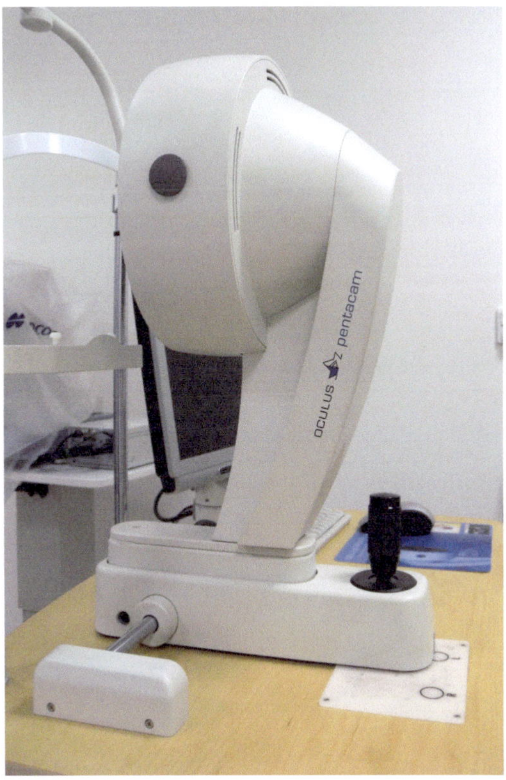

Fig. 1.19 Pentacam (Oculus) corneal topographer (side view)

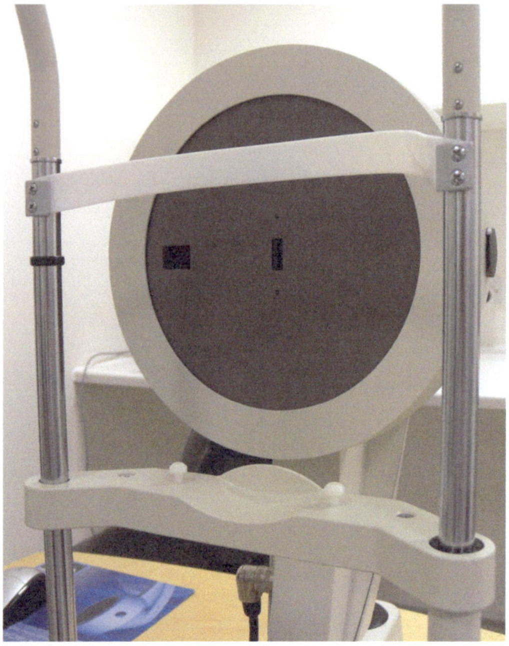

Fig. 1.20 Pentacam (Oculus) corneal topographer (patient view)

errors to more complex forms which have a more subtle effect on image quality.

Aberrometers were first used in astronomy where the effects of the earth's atmosphere degraded the images received from very distant objects. The principles have been adapted for in vivo analysis of the eye. Greater understanding of the effects of aberrations on image quality has assisted with the design of excimer laser ablation profiles and intraocular lenses.

A perfect lens refracts an incident ray of light, which is parallel to the optical axis, through the focal point to a point focus. If the lens or optical system is not perfect (i.e. contains aberrations), this will not be true, and the actual point at which an incident beam is focussed is shifted anteriorly or posteriorly (*focal shift*, the property measured). When the light beam is incident upon a different point on the lens, a corresponding focal shift is measured. Mapping the focal shift for each point on the lens gives an overall measurement of the

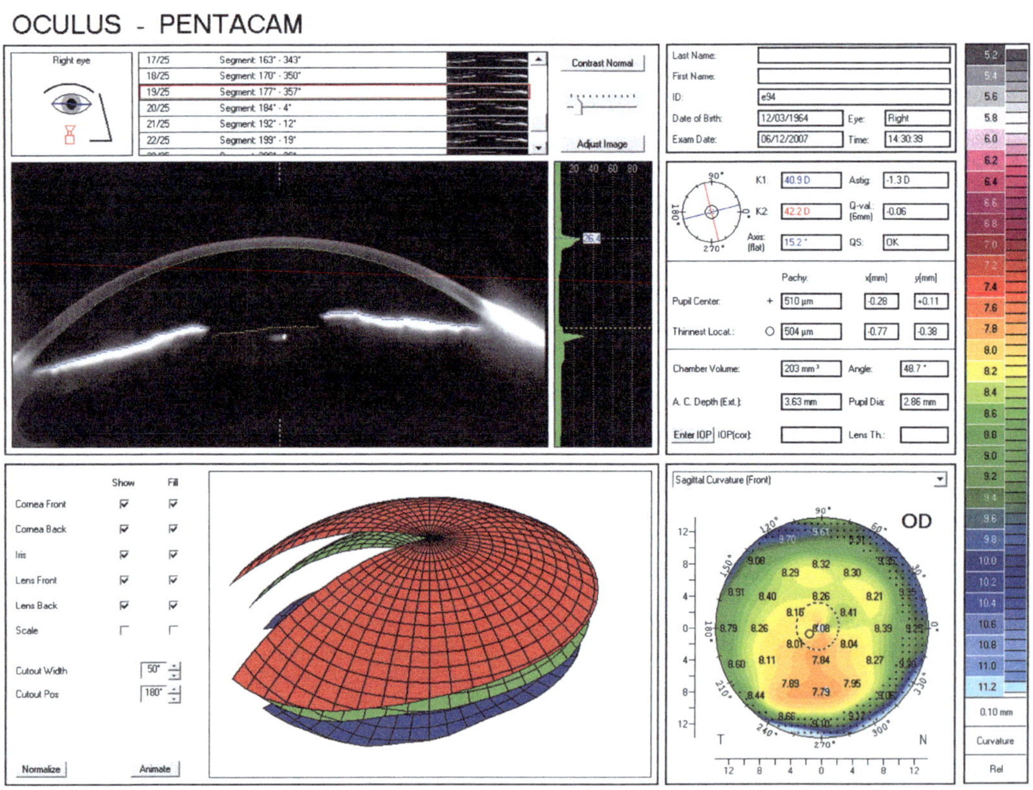

Fig. 1.21 Printout from Pentacam

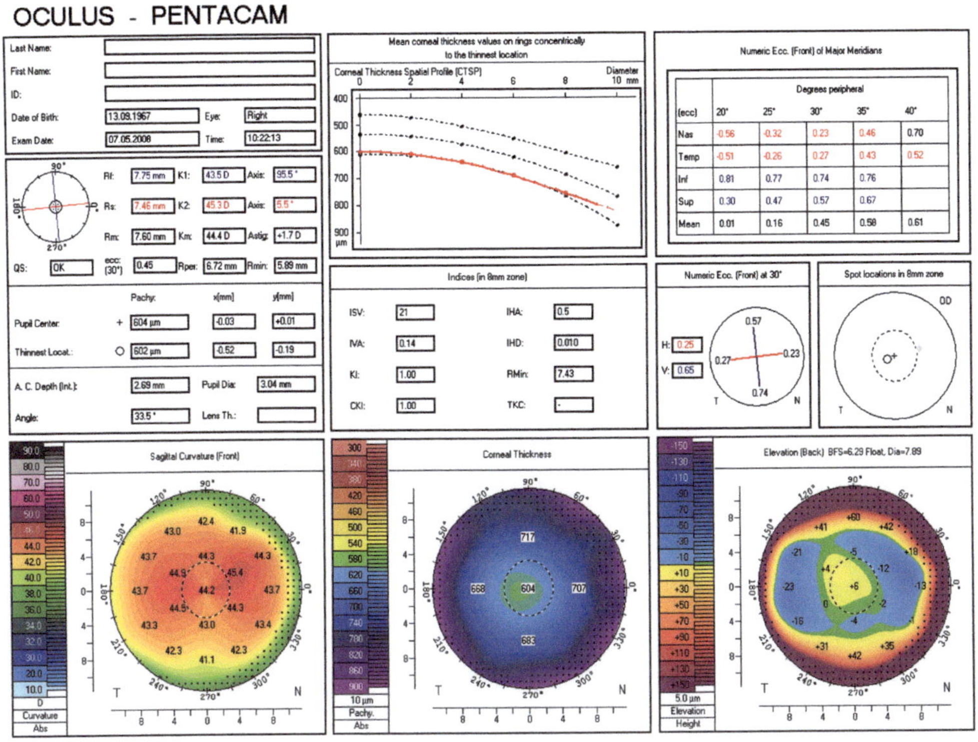

Fig. 1.22 Printout from Pentacam showing regular astigmatism

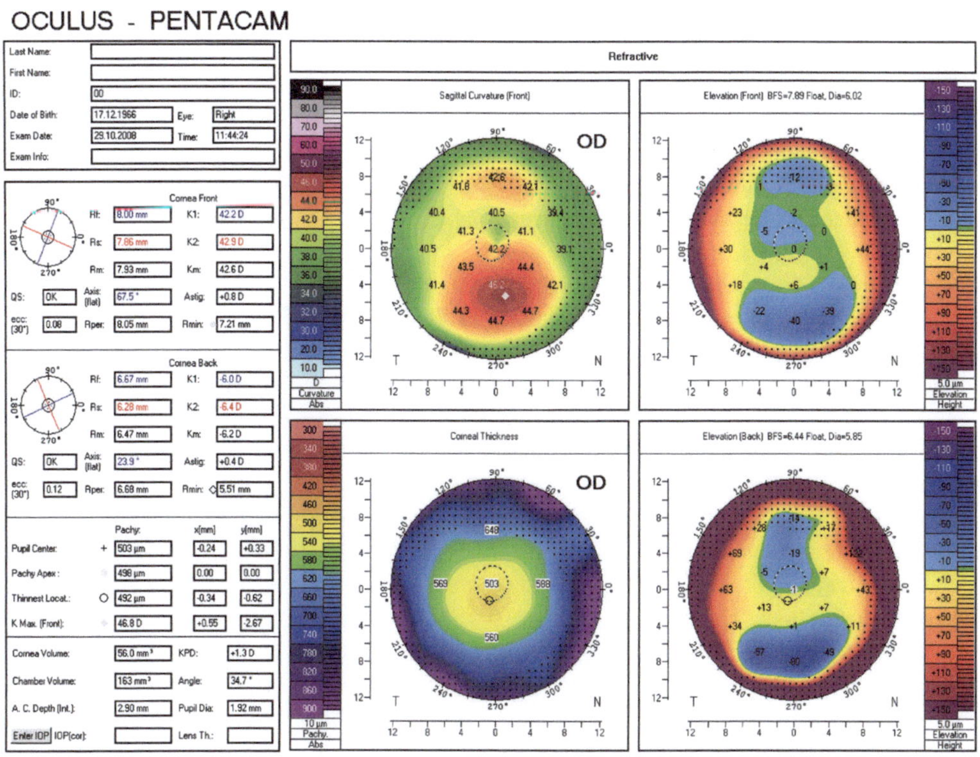

Fig. 1.23 Printout from Pentacam showing keratoconus Grade 1

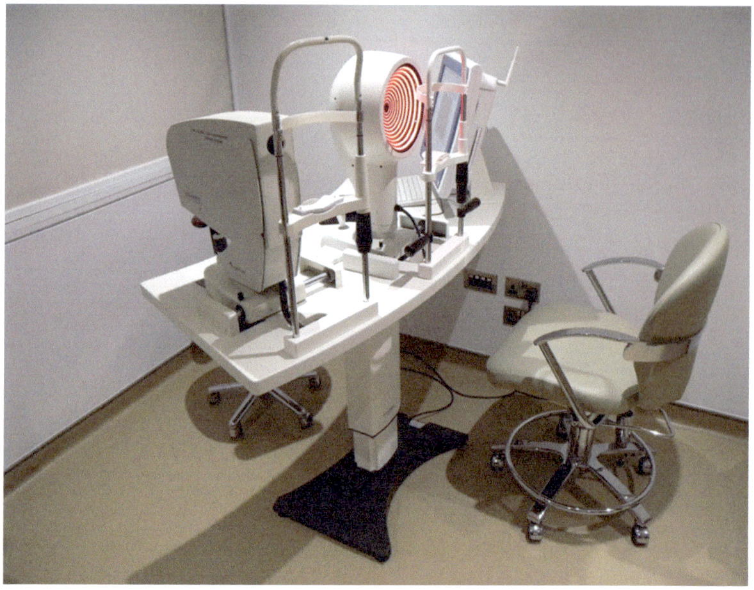

Fig. 1.24 Sirius (Schwind) corneal topographer with wavefront analyser

wavefront associated with that lens. This can be extended to an optical system, such as the eye.

The principle of the Hartmann-Shack aberrometer underlies most aberrometers in clinical use (e.g. Bausch&Lomb Zywave, AMO WaveScan, Schwind Wavefront Analyzer and Zeiss WASCA: Fig. 1.26). This involves projection of a narrow laser beam (850 nm for WASCA) with a known wavefront along the visual axis into the eye and detecting the reflected image at many points using an array of lenslets (each 500 μm in diameter) and a matrix of detectors. The composite of these reflected images is used to construct the reflected wavefront. Comparison of the perfect (i.e. aberration-free reference wavefront) and reflected wavefronts indicates the aberrations induced by the eye's optical elements.

The Tscherning principle (e.g. WaveLight Allegretto platform) is similar but uses multiple incident laser beams (660 nm) derived from a wide laser beam passing through a screen with a number of holes. This grid of spots is projected onto the retina, and the reflected spots are detected. The distortions in the pattern are used to derive the aberrations.

Ray-tracing analysis (e.g. Tracey Visual Function Analyzer) is an alternative method of assessing aberrations. Essentially, this involves projecting a laser beam (650 nm for Tracey VFA) onto the retina and recording its reflected image position. This is repeated for sufficient points to cover the pupil area (up to 256).

Statistical analysis of the reflected wavefront is expressed in terms of the mathematical equivalents of Zernike polynomials (Fig. 1.27). Aberrations of lower orders (defocus, astigmatism) and higher orders (spherical aberration, trefoil, coma and others) can all be analysed separately. On average, higher-order aberrations account for 4 % of total blur. Aberrations depend on pupil size, accommodation and target distance so it is important that aberrometers control for these.

1.5.10 Ocular Response Analyser (ORA)

The ocular response analyser is an instrument for assessing corneal hysteresis, a measure of viscous damping in the corneal tissue, that is, its tendency to absorb the energy of a deforming force. This originates in the viscoelastic nature of corneal tissue. A precisely metered pulse of air is applied to the vertex which causes a concave distortion of the corneal apex. Milliseconds later the pulse of air is stopped and the cornea resumes its natural shape, passing again through the applanated position to its resting shape. An optical detector system records when the cornea is in this applanated

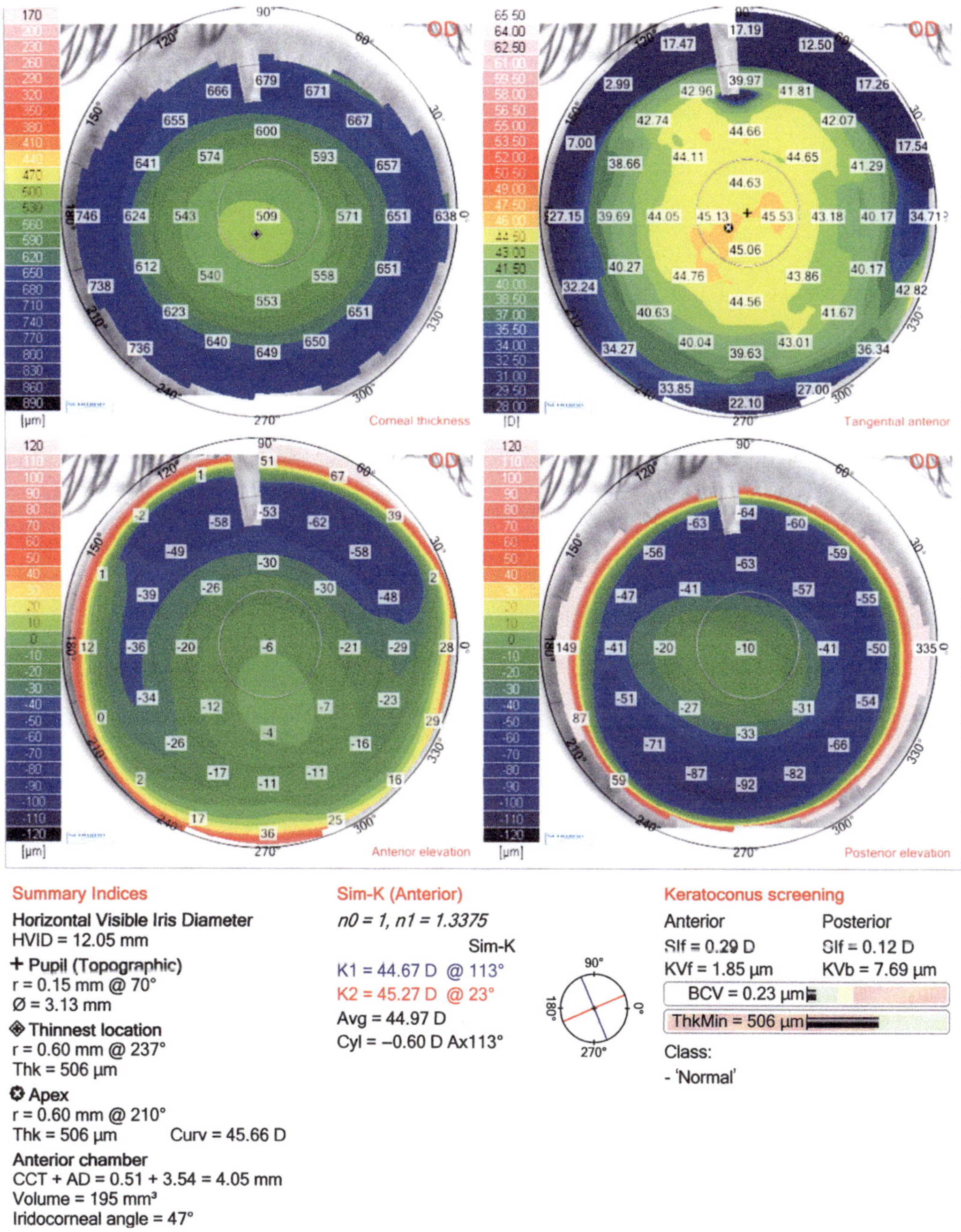

Fig. 1.25 Sirius printout

position during both deformation and recovery phases. The pressure of the air pulse is monitored throughout, and the two values at which the cornea is in the applanated position are recorded. The IOP is derived from these measured pressures by comparison against calibration values. The mean of the two IOP readings is the corrected IOP and the difference between them is the corneal hysteresis (in mmHg).

It is suggested that this is a more accurate way of measuring IOP as it is less affected by corneal factors (e.g. central corneal thickness) and prior

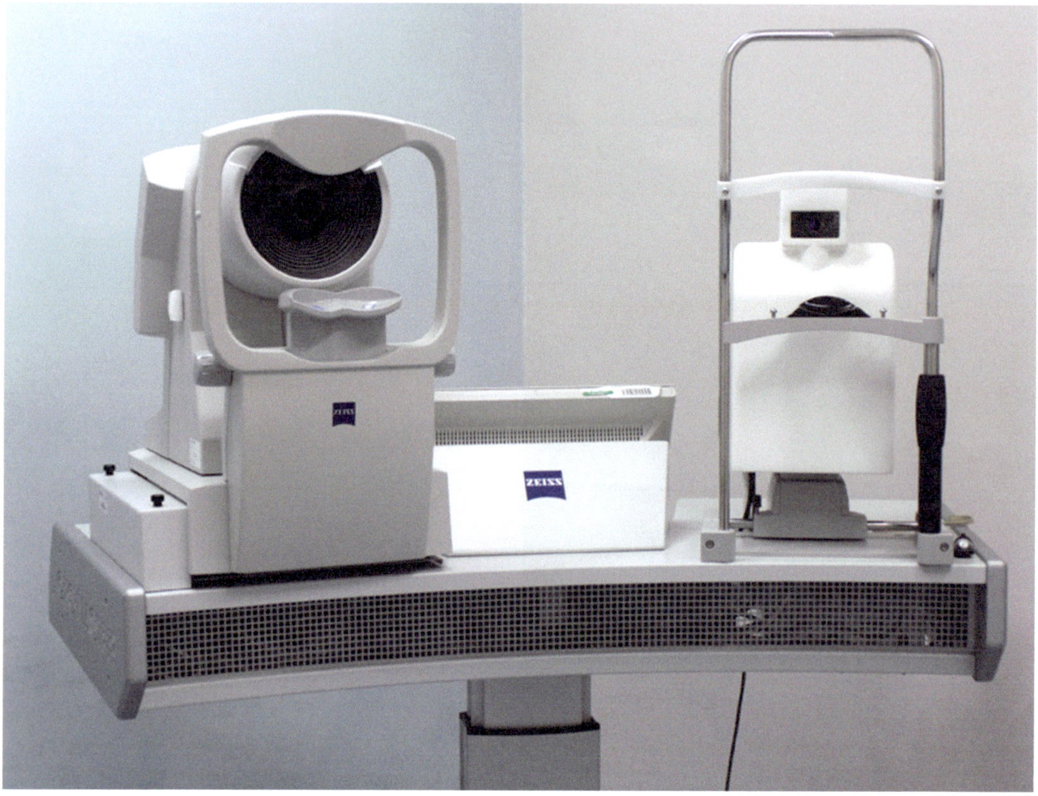

Fig. 1.26 Atlas (Zeiss) corneal topographer with WASCA wavefront analyser

surgery (LASIK or PKP) than other methods of tonometry, such as Goldman or pneumotonometry. It compensates for the biomechanical properties of the cornea as well as the central corneal thickness. It is a noncontact method and topical anaesthesia is not used.

The normal range for hysteresis is 8–16 mmHg. Low hysteresis values are seen in keratoconus, Fuchs's endothelial dystrophy and post-LASIK eyes. Eyes of older individuals also have a lower hysteresis value. High hysteresis values are seen in eyes with ocular hypertension.

Analysis of the readings obtained by the ORA also yields the Corneal Resistance Factor which is a measure of the combined effects of the viscous and elastic resistance encountered by the air puff while deforming the corneal surface (contrast hysteresis which is a measure of viscous damping alone). This is derived mathematically from the hysteresis value.

1.5.11 Optical Coherence Tomography (OCT)

OCT has been in use for some years for imaging the posterior segment and more recently for anterior segment imaging. There are several models in use, for example, the Zeiss Visante (Fig. 1.28).

For anterior segment OCT, a super-luminescent infrared (1310 nm) light source is used to acquire thousands of 'A-scans'. Analysis of the data enables a 'slice' through the anterior segment to be reconstructed at a resolution of 18 μm (Figs. 1.29 and 1.30). Built-in software allows accurate measurements to be made from the images. Tissue penetration is low (6 mm), and the incident beam is readily blocked by pigment so structures behind the iris are not visualised usefully. Penetration through corneal opacities is reasonable however so it can be used in patients with corneal scars to assess the remainder of the anterior segment which may not be easily assessed at the slit lamp. Angle

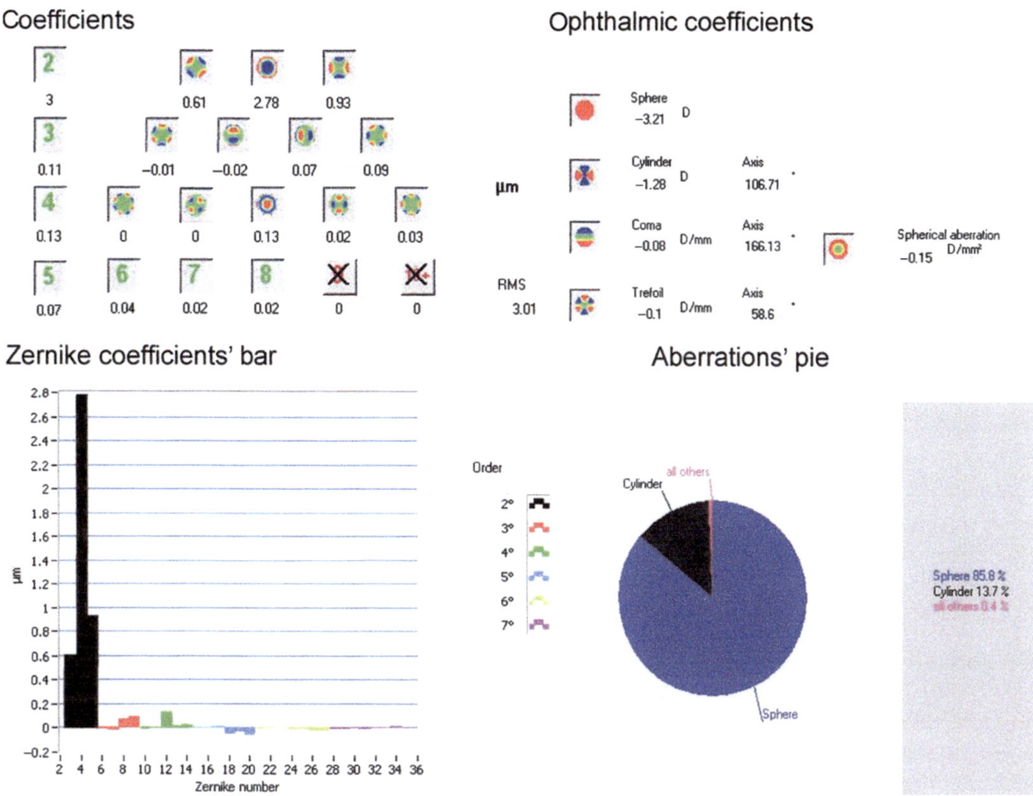

Fig. 1.27 Schwind wavefront printout

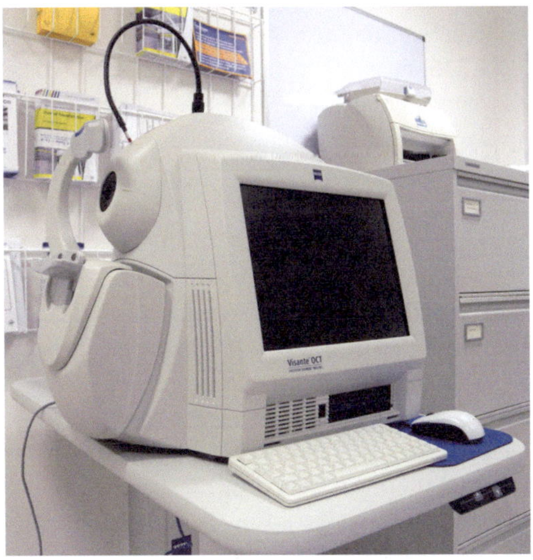

Fig. 1.28 Zeiss Visante anterior segment OCT

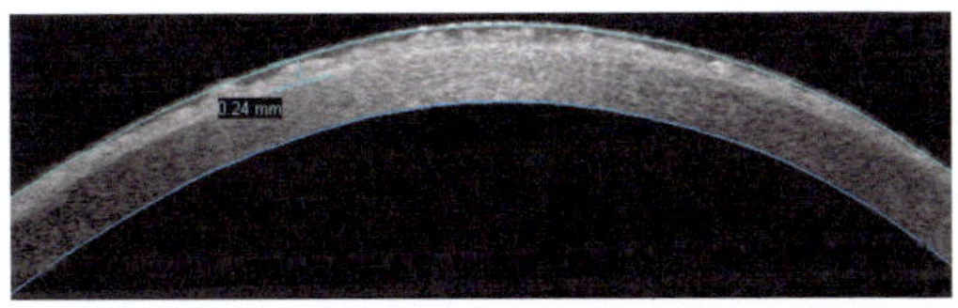

Fig. 1.29 Zeiss Visante OCT scan showing superficial anterior lamellar keratoplasty (SALK)

structures can be identified and the angle can be measured. Scan acquisition is very fast so patients with nystagmus can still be assessed in this way.

The latest generation of OCT instruments use spectral-domain or Fourier-domain scanning rather than the time-domain analysis used in the first generation of instruments. This allows faster scan acquisition (18–40,000 scans/s), and the shorter wavelength used gives greater resolution (5 µm). Reconstruction of data enables generation of simulated 3D images for ease of interpretation. One example of this is the OptoVue RTVue which uses an 830 nm light source and obtains 26,000 scans/s at a resolution of 5 µm.

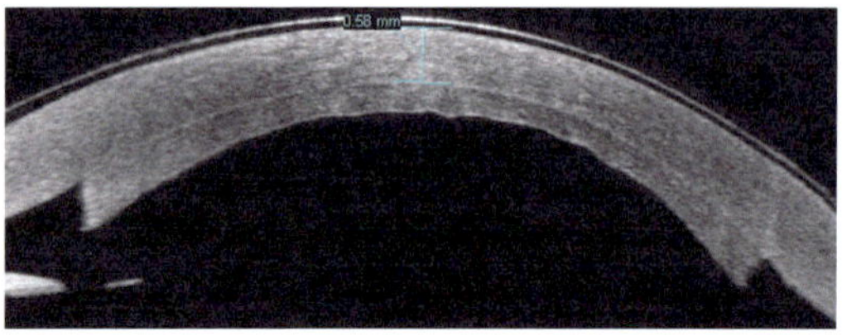

Fig. 1.30 Zeiss Visante OCT scan showing DSEK

1.5.12 Confocal Microscopy

This uses a pair of pinholes, a partial mirror and a condensing lens arranged so that a point source of light is focussed on the tissue under observation and the reflected image is focussed at an observing aperture. The two pinholes (one, the illuminating point, lies in front of a light source to provide a point source of light; the second, the observing point, is where the image is captured) are said to be confocal. Light reflected from nearby structures (different tissue depths or lying adjacent laterally) becomes sufficiently defocused at the observing aperture that it is not detected. In its simplest form only a single point of interest can be observed at any one time; in practice however an array of multiple points are used and scanned across the target at a rate which enables a composite image to be created. Some versions use a scanning slit for this rather than a pinhole. In this way the reflections and glare from structures around the point of interest which degrade the image of a light microscope and limit its resolution are avoided. Confocal microscopes in clinical use have a depth of field of 10–26 μm and a lateral resolution of 1–2 μm. This allows quantitative assessment of microscopic structures, particularly cells and nerves, and assessment of depth of visible structures, for example, scars or surgical planes.

The cornea can be imaged, for example, with the Nidek ConfoScan 4, which uses a scanning slit light source and reports a depth of field of 1 μm and lateral resolution of 0.6 μm. The appearance of the normal cornea and conjunctiva have been characterised along with characteristic findings in a range of pathologies, particularly acanthamoeba and fungal keratitis and various corneal dystrophies.

This technique is also employed in the Heidelberg Retinal Tomogram (HRT) with the Rostock Cornea Module, which uses a scanning diode laser at 670 nm. Image capture is very fast (24 ms) and eliminates artefact due to eye movement. Scans at different levels create images which are effectively optical sections and can be integrated to simulate a 3D image.

Serial scans over time can detect and measure changes in microstructure which is particularly useful. Characteristic changes apparent in corneal dystrophies have been described, for example, the liner branching structures in lattice dystrophy or the keratic precipitates and intercellular bright bodies seen during corneal graft rejection.

1.5.13 Specular Microscopy

Specular microscopy is the biomicroscopic examination of any corneal interface, especially the endothelium, using a reflected light beam. The image is obtained when the incident beam is reflected specularly (‘mirror like’), when the angle of incidence equals the angle of observation. The change in refractive index at the endothelium (corneal stroma $n = 1.376$, aqueous $n = 1.336$) means that enough light is reflected for the endothelium to be assessed, either qualitatively using the slit lamp or quantitatively using a specular microscope. At the slit lamp this is done by displacing the light beam and the eyepieces to the same angle either side of the midline (usually 60°). Observation is monocular using the high-magnification eyepiece at high magnification. The slit lamp is manoeuvred using the joystick towards the eye until the image of the endothelium is seen.

The specular microscope, for example, Topcon SP-3000P (Fig. 1.31) or Tomey EM-3000 (Fig. 1.32), employs a similar system, but computer control of the incident beam and image capture means that imaging can be automated and multiple images can be recorded. Inbuilt software can be used to identify individual cells for counting and analysis of cell density and morphology (Fig. 1.33). This gives a graphical output and allows serial measurements over time to be compared.

Sufficient light for examination of structures is only reflected at boundaries between structures which are sufficiently optically distinct. These are the air-tear film, tear film/epithelium and endothelium/aqueous interfaces. Intracorneal layers (i.e. between epithelium and Bowman's layer or between stroma and Descemet's membrane) also reflect a small amount of light but not enough for analysis.

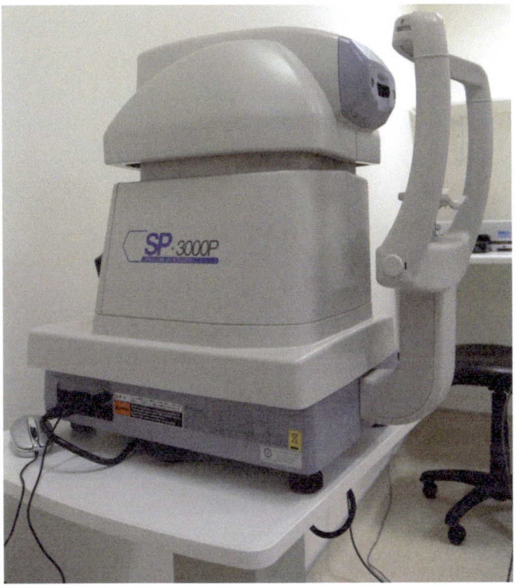

Fig. 1.31 SP 3000P (Topcon) specular microscope

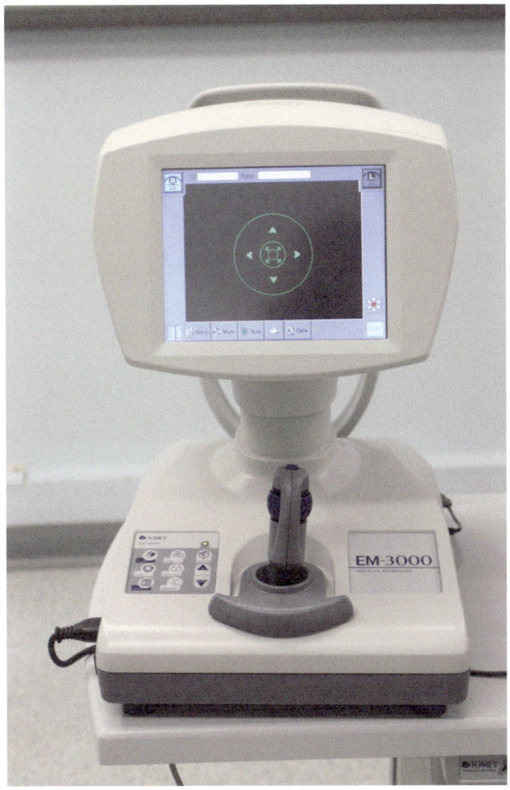

Fig. 1.32 EM-3000 (Tomey) specular microscope

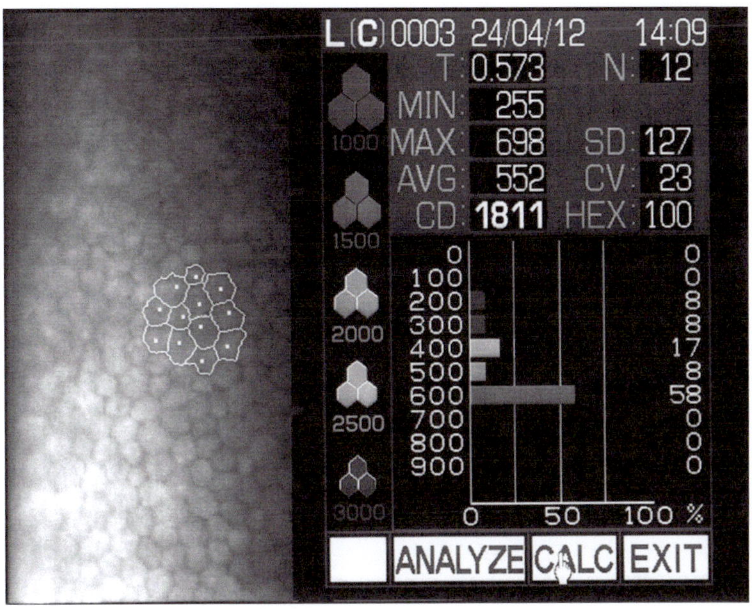

Fig. 1.33 SP 3000P printout

The quality of the reflected image depends on the width of the incident beam. A narrow beam will produce an image with reflected boundaries sufficiently separated so as not to interfere. A broad beam will produce broad images which overlap and degrade each other with a consequent loss of cellular definition. Automated systems overcome this difficulty by using a very narrow slit which scans across the desired area for adequate sampling without compromising image quality. The shallow depth of field of the microscope means that only the interface of interest is in focus at a given time.

Corneal oedema results in significant scattering of light rather than transmission and will impair image quality. Anterior chamber debris will result in some backscatter of the beam posterior to the endothelium which may make analysis of the images harder.

In young normal subjects the endothelial cell density is high (3,000–3,500 cells/mm^2) and their morphology and arrangement regular. In older normal subjects and corneas with endothelial dystrophies, this density will be less and cells are more varied in size and shape (polymegathism and pleomorphism), and arrangement will be more irregular. In Fuchs's endothelial dystrophy areas corresponding to guttata may be evident.

2 Ocular Surface and Reconstructive Surgery

2.1 Management of Corneal Foreign Bodies

Foreign bodies present a risk of infection and must be removed promptly. It is useful to establish the likely timescale and nature of the foreign body. The history will help to establish whether the object is likely to be superficial or penetrating.

Debris blown by the wind or falling on the eye is likely to cause a superficial foreign body which becomes attached via surface tension and adherent to the mucin layer and epithelial cells. Grinding injuries are common and may occur despite the user wearing a protective visor. The tiny metallic projectiles generated strike the eye at relatively low velocity and become embedded in the surface rather than penetrating. They tend to be hot and therefore often sterile, however, which allows them to fuse with superficial corneal tissue. A high-velocity fragment (such as is generated when chiselling stone or by metal-on-metal contact) would be more likely to penetrate through the cornea and results in an intraocular foreign body. This type of injury is outside the scope of this book and may require referral to a vitreo-retinal surgeon for further management. The palpebral conjunctiva including the fornices should be examined to exclude any other foreign bodies.

2.1.1 Superficial Foreign Bodies

Superficial foreign bodies (Fig. 2.1) can be removed with a sterile hypodermic needle or a low-speed burr. A cotton-tipped applicator is almost universally ineffective and should be avoided. This is because the foreign bodies will usually be too adherent and injudicious use is likely to cause an epithelial abrasion. Corneal foreign bodies in small children usually require a general anaesthesia for safe removal which can then be done using the operating microscope to ensure completeness. Clinical judgement should be applied however as a cooperative child with whom the clinician has a good rapport may allow removal under topical anaesthesia in the clinic.

Two different techniques can be used to remove a superficial foreign body.

2.1.1.1 The Needle Technique

The patient is positioned at the slit lamp and adequate topical analgesia is applied, for example, tetracaine or oxybuprocaine eye drops. Giving

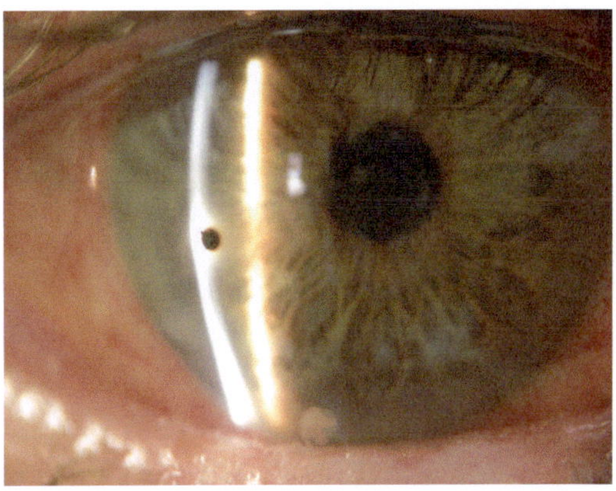

Fig. 2.1 Superficial metallic corneal foreign body

B. Zuberbuhler et al., *Corneal Surgery*,
DOI 10.1007/978-3-642-12502-7_2, © Springer-Verlag Berlin Heidelberg 2013

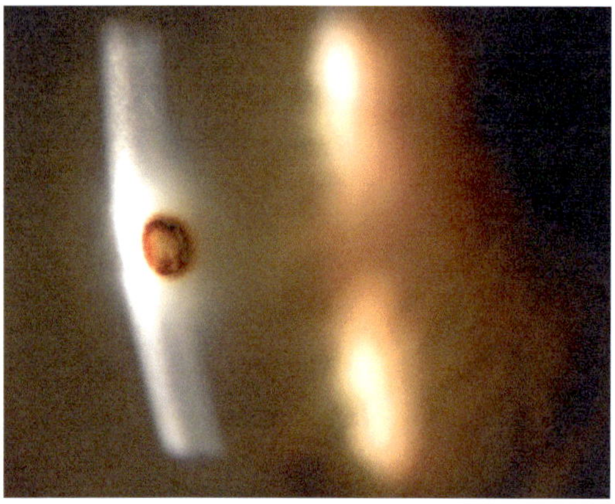

Fig. 2.2 Cornea with rost ring after removal of foreign body (same patient as Fig. 2.1)

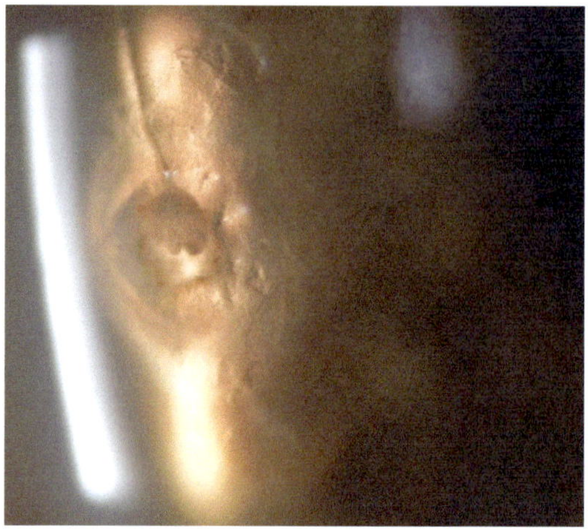

Fig. 2.3 Cornea after removal of foreign body and rost ring (same patient as Fig. 2.1)

topical anaesthetic to the fellow eye may aid fixation by reducing the urge to blink. A sterile 23G or 25G needle can be held directly or mounted on a 2 ml syringe to make it easier to manipulate. If the patient is unable to keep the eye open, the clinician should hold the lids open or insert a speculum. High or low magnification can be used as appropriate. The patient's gaze is directed so as to make the foreign body accessible and the edge of the bevel used to elevate the foreign body from the cornea. If a metallic foreign body has been present for 24 h or more, rust may be present which must also be removed (Fig. 2.2). This is done by using the edge of the bevel (or the needle tip with care) to get underneath the rust. A plane is sometimes easily found and the rust and metal lifts in one piece; if this is not possible, the fragments of rust must be swept from the cornea using the side of the bevel tip. This often leaves a small crater in the stroma which will remodel (Fig. 2.3). All foreign material must be removed to prevent it forming a focus for infection. If it is not possible at the first attempt, the patient should be prescribed a topical antibiotic and asked to return in 3–4 days for further debridement. This provides prophylaxis against infection and the foreign material may loosen so that removal is easier at the next attempt.

2.1.1.2 The Burr Technique

The burr most commonly used has an internal motor which rotates a sterile abrasive tip. Preparation is as above and the side of the burr is used to remove the foreign body. This is most effective for embedded foreign bodies, particularly if there is a fragmented rust ring. Particular care must be taken if the patient has had previous LASIK, especially if the foreign body is near the flap edge as there have been reports of the burr lifting and damaging the flap. Care must also be exercised with patients who have had a previous corneal graft to avoid inducing a dehiscence of the graft-host interface. Once all foreign material has been removed, the patient is prescribed a broad-spectrum topical antibiotic and advised regarding analgesia. Shields or pads are not essential and if removal is complete routine follow-up is not needed.

2.1.2 Embedded Foreign Bodies

If a foreign body is embedded in corneal stroma (e.g. thorn), it may be difficult to determine how deep it has penetrated. Seidel's test with 2 % fluorescein may help identify the presence of an aqueous leak, and the anterior segment must be examined carefully for signs of intraocular perforation or other associated injuries. Sometimes, a CT scan is performed to locate or exclude (metallic) intraocular foreign bodies.

Foreign body removal in the operating theatre using the microscope is recommended in case a perforation which requires suturing or gluing is identified after removal of the foreign body. Sub-Tenon's or peribulbar anaesthesia may be preferred for this. The foreign body should be withdrawn back along its original trajectory and sent for microbiological analysis and culture since the risk of infection is significant. A bandage contact lens may be placed depending on the nature of injury and the treatment required. A broad-spectrum topical antibiotic and cycloplegia are given, and the patient is reviewed in the clinic 5–7 days later.

Any suspicion of infection merits prompt scraping for microbiological analysis and intensive topical antibiotics to prevent abscess formation. If the foreign body was organic material (e.g. thorn or wood) or dirty, fungal infection should be considered and treatment adjusted appropriately.

The major long-term complication is scar formation which may be visually significant if it affects the visual axis. Management for corneal scarring is considered in later chapters.

2.2 Management of Corneal Perforations

2.2.1 Gluing

Micro-perforations may be observed and managed expectantly as most will self-seal within 24 h. A bandage contact lens may be placed to aid this.

Small corneal perforations (<1 mm) may be successfully managed with tissue glues. The two forms in common use are *N*-butyl-2-cyanoacrylate preparations and fibrin-based glues (e.g. Tisseel). Cyanoacrylate setting is triggered by contact with fluid and air. The surface to which cyanoacrylate is to be applied must be dry as any fluid at the glue-tissue interface will prevent proper adhesion and must be free from epithelium as this will slough off and cause the glue to dehisce. The glue sets with an exothermic reaction which cauterises tissue and causes tissue contraction which helps to close the perforation. Application in the operating theatre under the microscope is preferred, but it can be done under aseptic conditions at the slit lamp if necessary.

2.2.1.1 Cyanoacrylate

Topical anaesthetic is given (e.g. tetracaine 1 %). If infection is suspected, swabs and/or scrape may be taken at this time. Epithelium and debris are cleared from the cornea around the perforation and the size of the defect reassessed. The area is dried carefully using cellulose sponge spears.

Various techniques can be used to apply the glue:

- A 25G needle is fitted to the glue sachet and a small meniscus of glue is raised at the bevel. The needle is then used to apply a small quantity of glue directly onto the perforation. The tissue reaction as the glue sets can be seen in the area immediately surrounding the perforation. Small amounts of glue are added until a sufficient area has been treated. If a number of droplets of glue are required, the needle may need to be exchanged as it is prone to blockage. A bandage contact lens (silicon hydrogel 14 mm) is placed and topical broad-spectrum antibiotic (ofloxacin) is given at the end of the procedure. The patient is prescribed regular antibiotic drops and reviewed the next day.
- Using a small (3 mm) punch biopsy trephine, a sterile plastic disc is cut from a clear drape. This is attached to the tip of a cellulose sponge spear using a small blob of chloramphenicol ointment or other gel (Fig. 2.4). A small drop of glue is then placed onto the disc. When this is inverted onto the perforation, the glue and its plastic carrier will attach and will come away from the sponge spear easily (Fig. 2.5). For a larger perforation this can be repeated with several adjacent glue/disc units. Again, once the perforation is sealed, a bandage contact lens is placed for comfort and to reduce the risk of disc displacement, and topical broad-spectrum antibiotic drops are given.
- Glue can also be used to reinforce an area of peripheral ulceration or guttering. Glue is drawn up into an insulin syringe from which it is applied accurately into the area of corneal thinning. Again, a bandage contact lens is placed and topical antibiotics prescribed.

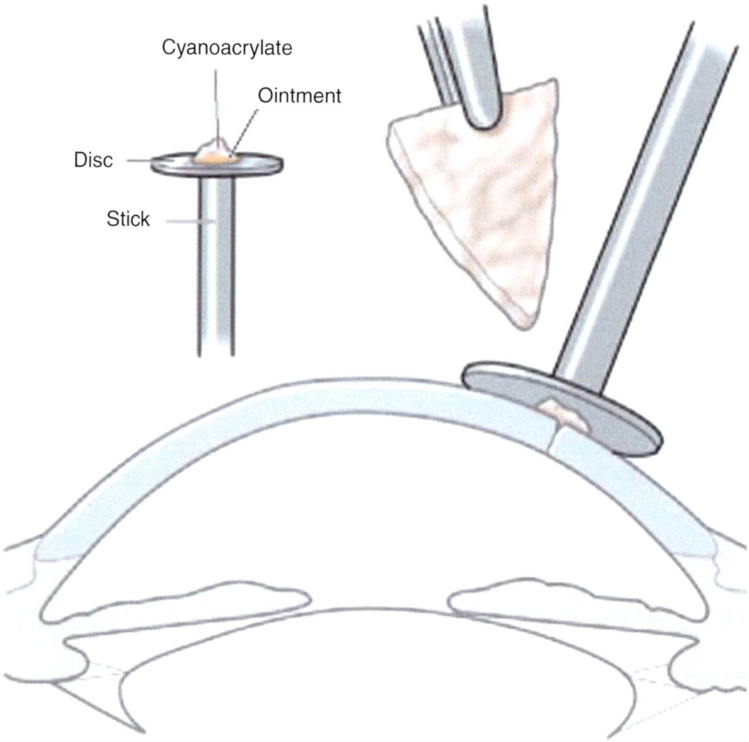

Fig. 2.4 Illustration of corneal gluing

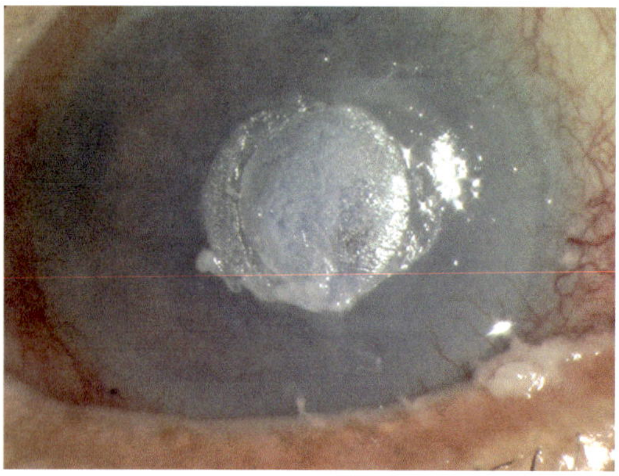

Fig. 2.5 Glued cornea with plastic disc

The glue will spontaneously detach after about a week (although it sometimes takes longer), by which time it is hoped that the underlying tissue will have healed. If it has not healed, the gluing procedure can be repeated. If it was initially anticipated that a tectonic graft would be needed for definitive closure, the gluing buys time to quieten the eye, treat any infection and obtain graft material. However, any glue should be removed at about 4 weeks to reduce the risk of infection and vascularisation.

2.2.1.2 Fibrin Glue

Fibrin glue is manufactured from the cryoprecipitate obtained from pooled donated blood products. Components are prepared into two syringes and kept separate until needed. One component is a fibrinogen preparation; the other is a thrombin solution for activating the fibrinogen. The contents of both syringes are applied simultaneously onto the target tissue; as they mix, fibrinogen is converted to fibrin and a plug forms. This is effective at sealing small perforations but dissolves more rapidly than cyanoacrylate.

2.2.2 Suturing

A perforation larger than 1–2 mm may be managed by placing one or more corneal sutures (Fig. 2.6). Prolapsed iris may temporarily tamponade the wound and has to be replaced before suturing (Fig. 2.7). A successful outcome is more likely if the perforation is linear (e.g. after sharp trauma) than round (e.g. a large perforated ulcer) as closing a round defect in this way will induce tension and striae. Interrupted 10/0 nylon

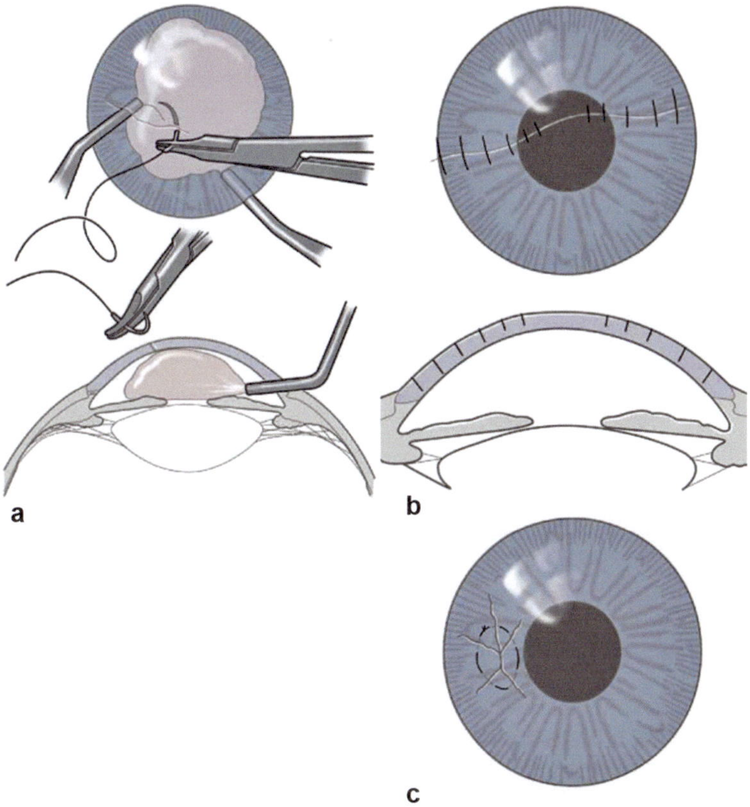

Fig. 2.6 Illustration of suture techniques for traumatic corneal perforation. (**a**) Use of viscoelastic to reform anterior chamber; (**b**) appropriate length and depth of sutures, avoiding visual axis; (**c**) technique for stellate wound

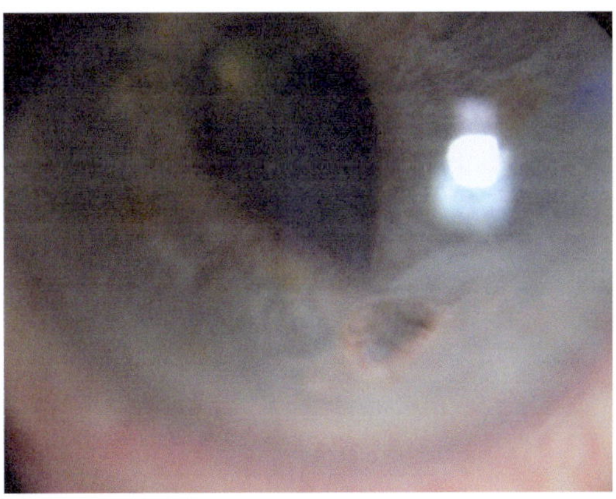

Fig. 2.7 Corneal perforation with iris prolapsed/tamponade

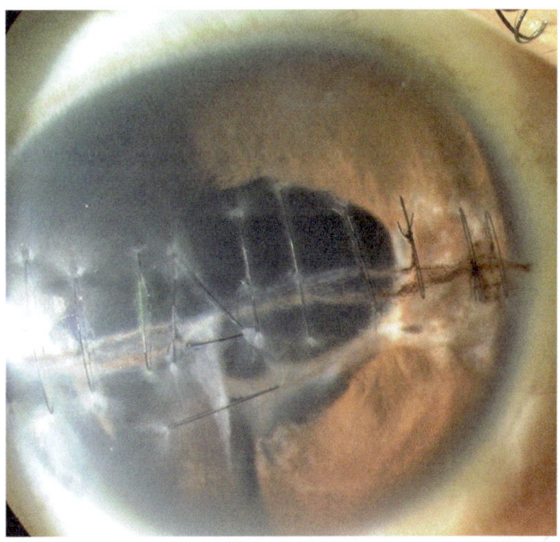

Fig. 2.8 Corneal repair with interrupted sutures 3 months following penetrating injury

sutures are preferred. If possible placing sutures in the visual axis should be avoided. Perforations larger than 3 mm (Figs. 2.8 and 2.9) should be sutured under general anaesthesia (risk of expulsive haemorrhage). An iris defect or iridodialysis may be repaired at the same time (Figs. 2.10 and 2.11). Very severe ocular injuries, for example, from a bomb blast, with multiple large perforations and iris and vitreous prolapse have to be consented with a view to enucleation (Fig. 2.12).

2.2.3 Tectonic Graft

If the perforation is too large for glue or fails to heal satisfactorily after gluing, it may be necessary to repair the defect with a full-thickness or lamellar patch graft. All attempts must be made to address any inflammation (systemic steroids in melting corneas) and infection before grafting is undertaken, although this may not be possible if the need for grafting is urgent. It may be possible to repair a small peripheral corneal or corneo-scleral defect while completely avoiding the visual axis. Repair of a larger defect may result in scarring over the visual axis. In this case a larger

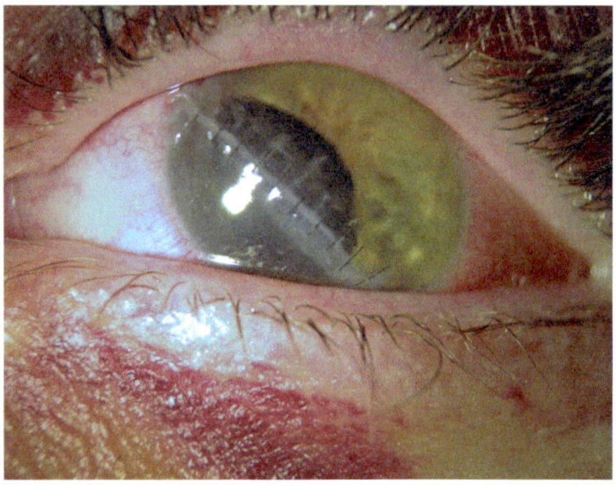

Fig. 2.9 Corneal repair with interrupted sutures 2 weeks postoperative, VA 6/24

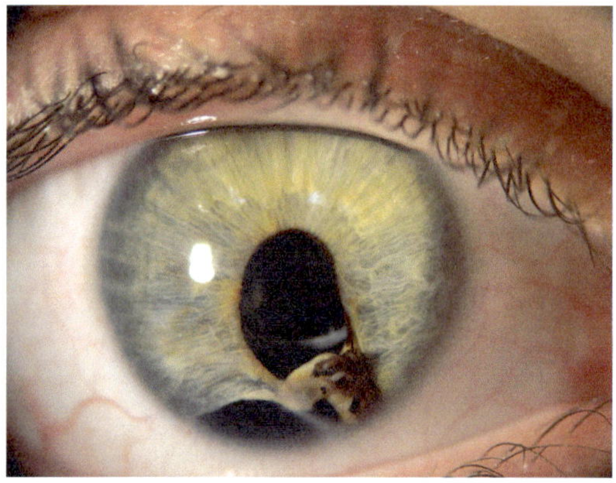

Fig. 2.11 Traumatic iris defect, old

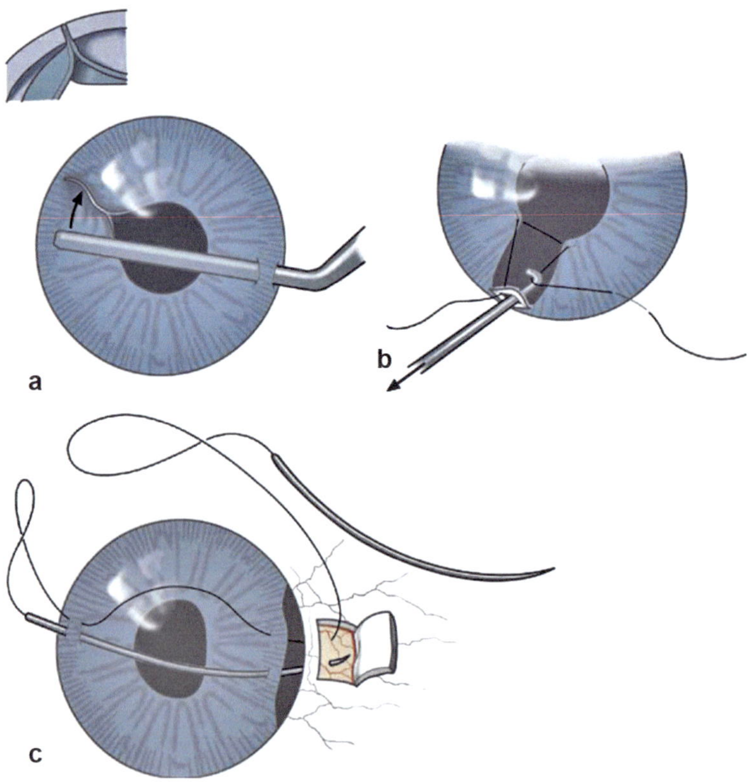

Fig. 2.10 Illustration of management of iris reconstruction and iridodialysis repair. (**a**) Sweeping prolapsed iris away from a corneal wound; (**b**) McCannel suture to close an iris defect; (**c**) repair of iridodialysis

area of cornea should be replaced which incorporates the visual axis into the graft. Close monitoring is essential to watch for signs of melting, infection or rejection.

2.3 Pterygium

Pterygium is a triangular- or wing-shaped proliferation of fibrovascular tissue originating from conjunctiva and subconjunctival tissue propagating across the limbus onto the cornea (Fig. 2.13). It is more common nearer the equator, especially in countries between 0° and 30° of latitude, and is linked to chronic exposure to sunlight, particularly UVB radiation. Incidence varies from 0.3 to 29 %. Reasons for presenting include cosmetic (most common), ocular surface discomfort and visual impairment, either due to induced astigmatism (usually with the rule) or rarely obstruction of the visual axis. Surgery may be offered for any of these reasons although astigmatism and visual obstruction are most readily addressed. Many patients still have residual symptoms of ocular surface discomfort after surgery, even if successful (Figs. 2.14 and 2.15).

2.3.1 Surgical Removal

Surgery is performed under sub-Tenon's, peribulbar or GA. An occlusive contact lens or sponge disc may be placed on the cornea to prevent retinal phototoxicity. A 7/0 silk stay suture can be placed through superior cornea for easy mobilisation of the eye.

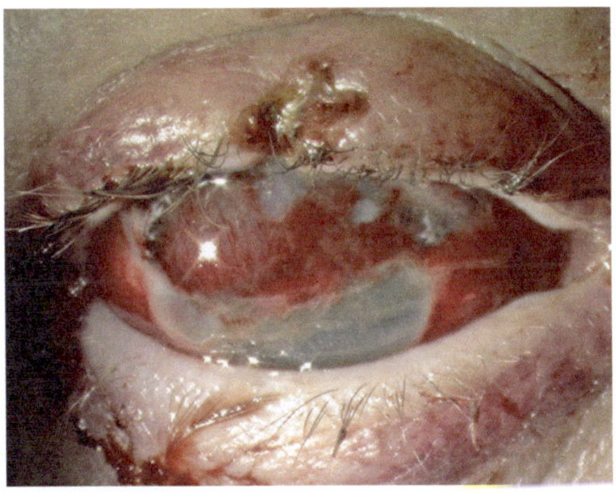

Fig. 2.12 Severe globe rupture following bomb blast in 2008 in the Middle East war zone

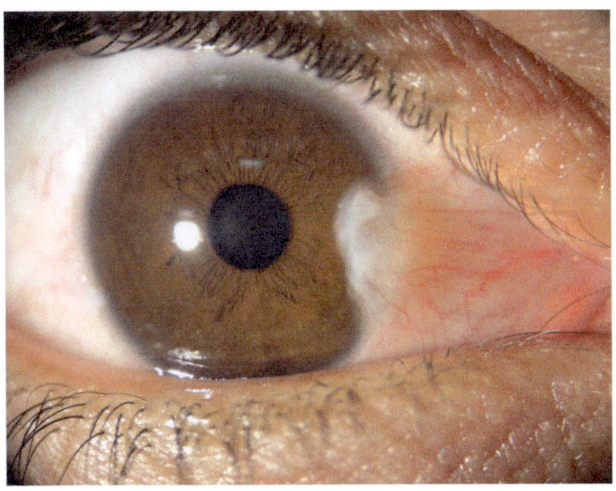

Fig. 2.13 Medium-sized pterygium

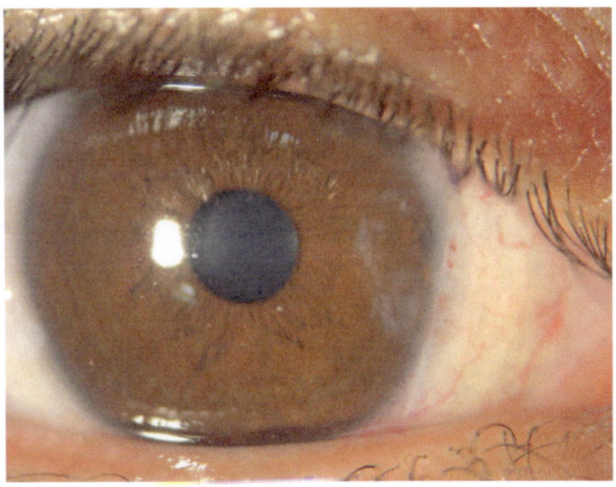

Fig. 2.14 Two months after pterygium repair with autograft (same patient as Fig. 2.13; front)

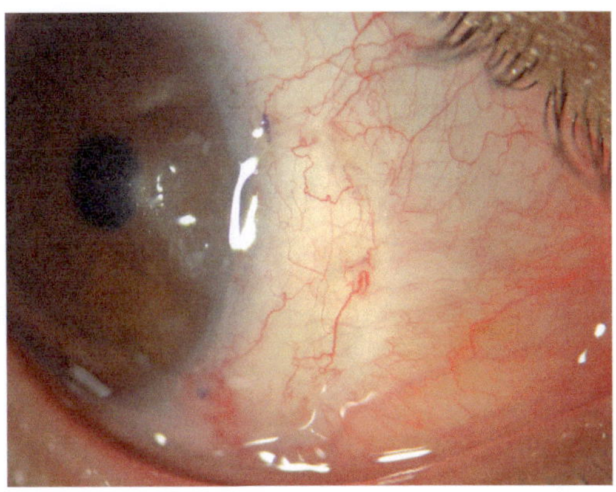

Fig. 2.15 Two months after pterygium repair with autograft (same patient as Fig. 2.13; graft)

2.3.1.1 Peeling Technique (for Primary Pterygium)

A limbal cut separates the head and body of the pterygium. The head of the pterygium is grasped with forceps at the limbus and firm traction is applied tangentially to pull the head away from the cornea towards the corneal centre (Fig. 2.16). The abnormal tissue should come away cleanly from the cornea, although it may be necessary to remove any small areas of residual tissue on the corneal surface. Blunt dissection beneath the pterygium directed peripherally is then used to free up all the abnormal tissue down to bare sclera. The pterygium is usually quite distinct from normal conjunctival tissue and the margins should be evident (preserve as much healthy conjunctiva as possible). The resulting conjunctival gap is then covered with a conjunctival autograft (see below).

2.3.1.2 Lamellar Dissection Technique

The head is dissected from the cornea using a hockey stick blade (Fig. 2.16). The correct plane of separation may be difficult to identify clearly, and care must be taken not to dissect too deeply. When the head is free the body can be dissected with scissors and the pterygium freed at its edges. This approach is more likely to induce postoperative astigmatism, especially if the pterygium had encroached close to the visual axis.

2.3.1.3 Conjunctival Autograft

After removal of a small pterygium, the conjunctiva can often be closed directly. Larger defects must be covered with conjunctival tissue from elsewhere. A conjunctival autograft is the most physiological approach to this, and a free graft is taken from the superior-temporal bulbar conjunctiva. The area to be covered is measured orthogonally with callipers for its greatest linear dimensions

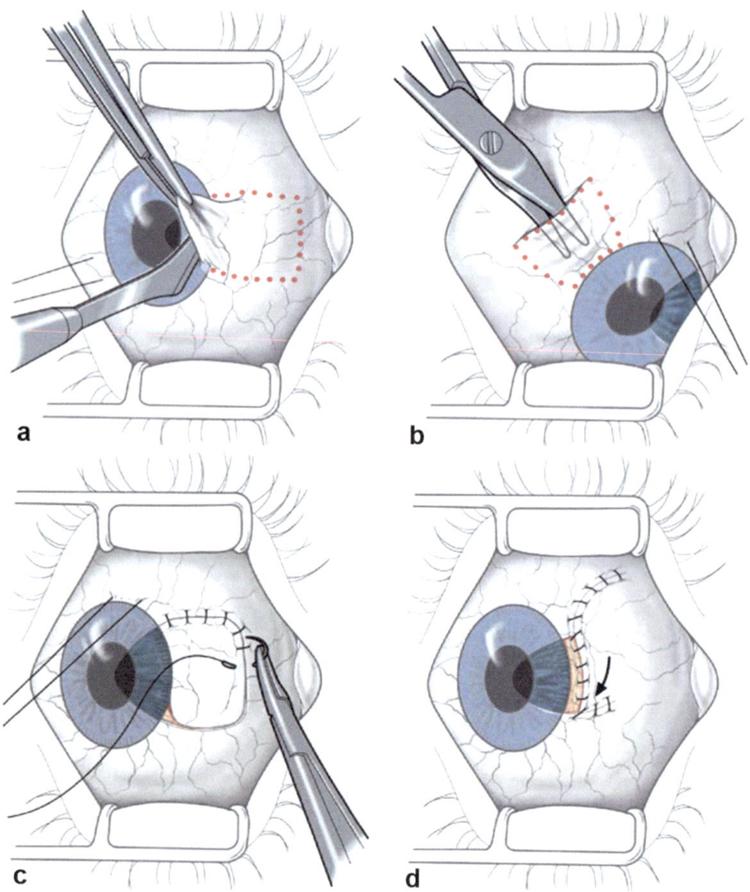

Fig. 2.16 Illustration of pterygium excision with autograft. (**a**) Excising the pterygium; (**b**) preparing the conjunctival autograft; (**c**) securing the free conjunctival autograft; (**d**) alternative method of covering bared sclera with a conjunctival rotation flap

and a slightly oversized area of conjunctiva marked with ink at the host site. A conjunctival graft which is too small may result in it being under tension, risking graft dehiscence or tethering to the caruncle which may limit abduction.

As most host sites show healthy normal tissues, a direct separation of conjunctiva and Tenon capsule is possible with fine Westcott scissors. Some surgeons prefer to inject 1 % lignocaine with adrenaline on a 25G needle under the conjunctiva with the aim to raise a bleb. This bleb is then enlarged and massaged across the marked area to begin the separation of conjunctiva away from Tenon's capsule. Westcott scissors are then introduced into this space, and the two layers are separated by snipping rather than spreading to cleanly separate fine adhesions. The whole area is undermined before the edges are cut. The graft is cut free around its edge and slid around onto the bared medial sclera paying attention to its orientation. A marker may be placed to aid orientation and prevent the graft being applied upside down. We favour a larger ink mark at one corner but a suture may also be used. In addition, the limbal site of the graft should be oriented to the limbal site of the bare sclera (stem cell support for the corneal wound healing). The corners and sides are secured with interrupted vicryl 8/0, 9/0 or 10/0 sutures, which must also anchor the graft to the sclera, usually done at the limbus only. Alternatively, the edges of the graft can be secured with fibrin glue, and a large bandage contact lens (18–20 mm) can be placed for comfort and protection.

Conjunctival autograft reduces the rate of recurrence (7.9 %, pooled data) compared to excision only (37 %, Youngson) and avoids the risks associated with mitomycin. Amniotic membrane has been used in place of a conjunctival autograft but was also associated with high recurrence rates.

2.3.1.4 Follow-Up Plan

Postoperatively preservative-free dexamethasone 0.1 % (6×/day) and chloramphenicol (qds) eye drops are given (Table 2.1). Oral diclofenac 50 mg tds or paracetamol 500 mg qds can be added for analgesia. Review is usually at 1 day, 1 week, 1 month and 3 months.

2.3.1.5 Complications

Buttonhole of the graft, although it is not clear whether repair of buttonholes with 10/0 vicryl is beneficial. Some surgeons do not consider holes in the graft as a disadvantage and occasionally deliberately 'mesh' the graft with small snips if the fit is too small for the bare sclera site, with good outcomes. Other intraoperative complications include inadvertent inversion of the graft, globe perforation, bleeding and medial rectus injury. Postoperative complications include pyogenic granuloma, postoperative astigmatism (rare), graft dehiscence, discomfort, dellen and persistent epithelial defects. Late complications are pterygium recurrence, graft contracture and limitation of abduction by tethering of scar tissue.

2.3.2 Antimetabolites

As an adjunct to surgical excision or as an alternative to conjunctival graft, mitomycin C (MMC) reduces the rate of pterygium recurrence. It can be applied intraoperatively to the sclera after pterygium excision via sponges soaked in solutions of 0.01–0.04 %. The most common approach is 0.02 % for 3 min followed by copious

Table 2.1 Review plan and treatment after pterygium surgery

Visit	Prescription	Examination
Preoperative		Photo
Day of surgery	G Dexamethasone-N 6×/day for 4 weeks PO Paracetamol 500 mg Tabl 4×/day for 1 week	
1–2 days (optional)		Positioning
1 week		Remove CL
1 month	G Dexamethasone 3×/day for 1 week G Dexamethasone 2×/day for 1 week G Dexamethasone 1×/day for 1 week	IOP (steroids)
3–6 months	None	Photo

irrigation. Alternatively MMC 0.02 % eye drops can be given postoperatively, usually qds for 10 days. MMC is associated with rare late complications including limbal stem cell failure, glaucoma, iritis, corneal oedema, scleral necrosis, infectious scleritis, perforations and endophthalmitis. It is usually reserved for very active pterygia or recurrences.

2.4 Phototherapeutic Keratectomy

Phototherapeutic keratectomy (PTK) is the superficial ablation of corneal tissue with the excimer laser to treat pathologies affecting the corneal epithelium or anterior corneal stroma. It is most applicable to disorders limited to the anterior 10–20 % of stroma.

2.4.1 Indications and Contraindications

2.4.1.1 Indications

- Recurrent corneal erosion following trauma
- Dystrophies of epithelium and Bowman's layer (e.g. recurrent corneal erosions, map-dot-fingerprint dystrophy, mild band keratopathy) affecting vision
- Superficial corneal scars and band-shaped corneal degeneration (Fig. 2.17), vernal plaque in adults

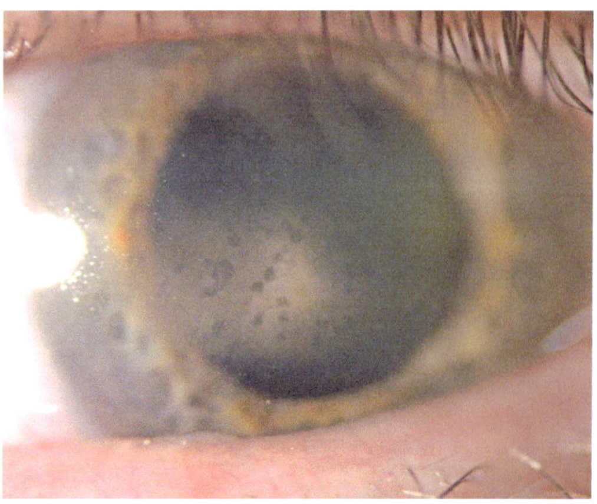

Fig. 2.17 Band keratopathy

- Anterior stromal dystrophies (e.g. Reis-Bücklers, Thiel-Behnke (honeycomb) dystrophies, Granular type I dystrophy)

2.4.1.2 Contraindications

- Deep stromal lesions, dense band keratopathy
- Significant corneal thinning
- Neurotrophic cornea, lagophthalmos
- Severe keratoconjunctivitis sicca
- Severe blepharitis
- Any corneal infection

2.4.2 Technique

Topical anaesthetic (e.g. tetracaine) and povidone iodine are applied, the eye is draped and a speculum placed. The patient is placed supine beneath the excimer laser. The epithelium is removed by debridement using cellulose spears. Any small areas difficult to remove can be cleared by brushing with a hockey stick-type blade. If the laser has a slit-lamp attachment, this can be used to assess for any remaining islands of epithelium which must be cleared. Some surgeons prefer to remove the epithelium with the excimer laser (Trans-PTK: 50 μm depth).

The laser is then used to ablate a uniform profile over as large an area of cornea as possible (usually 6.5–8 mm) centred on the pupil. The depth of ablation (Table 2.2) will depend on the pathology being treated; as an example for recurrent corneal erosions, 10 μm deep across the cornea is appropriate. If there are marked irregularities, masking fluid (e.g. carboxymethylcellulose 0.5 %) can be used to fill in 'valleys' and leave 'peaks' exposed for ablation. The aim is to remove the least amount of tissue possible while removing as much opacity as possible (Fig. 2.18). For localised or raised lesions, the ablating laser beam may be steered manually by the joystick. At the end of the procedure, preservative-free chloramphenicol eye drops are given and a bandage contact lens is placed.

Patient information should include:

- There will be a noise and it will smell.
- A moderate pain will start after a view hours.

Table 2.2 Review plan and treatment after pterygium surgery

Corneal lesion	Depth of ablation (after removal of epithelium)
Recurrent corneal erosion	6–10 µm
Band keratopathy	25 µm
Corneal dystrophy	25–50 µm
Trans-PTK	Add 50 µm to above depths

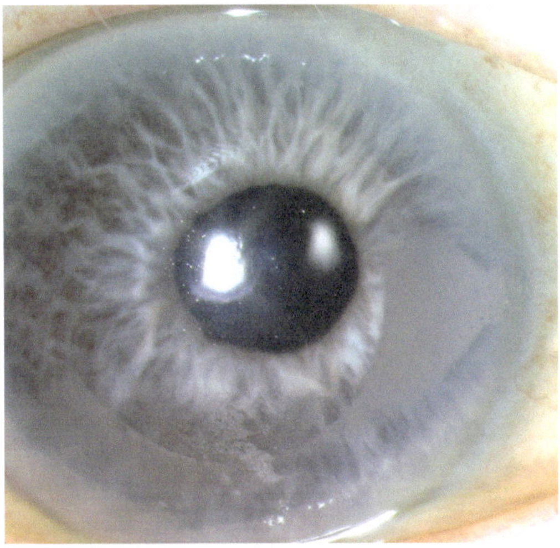

Fig. 2.18 One week after phototherapeutic keratoplasty (PTK) for band keratopathy

- Patient should use sun glasses (postoperative photophobia).
- PTK can induce a hyperopic refractive change or irregular astigmatism.
- There is the possibility of recurrences and scars.

2.4.3 Aftercare

A typical postoperative treatment consists of topical antibiotics (e.g. chloramphenicol qds), corticosteroids (e.g. dexamethasone qds) and anti-inflammatory eye drops (diclofenac tds), all for 1–2 weeks. Lubricant eye drops (e.g. Hypromellose qds) and mydriatic eye drops (e.g. cyclopentolate bd) can be added. The patient is reviewed after 2 days for signs of infection and again 1–2 weeks later. The contact lens can be removed after corneal re-epithelialisation. Topography and refraction should be performed after 4 weeks. PTK can be repeated for recurrence of dystrophy.

2.4.4 Complications

- No effect, especially for recurrent corneal erosion.
- Hyperopic shifts are common as a result from flattening of the central cornea, especially with deeper ablations (rule of thumb: 15 µm = 1 D (dioptre)). Irregular astigmatism may develop if the ablation was decentred or if inadequate masking was used.
- Pain; regular analgesia should be advised.
- Delayed epithelialisation with risk of infection: The bandage contact lens and frequent lubrication may aid re-epithelialisation. Punctal plugs may be considered in patients with severe dry eyes.
- Reactivation of a herpes simplex virus keratitis (HSK) is possible from stimulation of the corneal nerve plexus by the ablation. Where possible, treatment of patients with previous HSK should be avoided. If such patients are treated, prophylactic pre- and postoperative acyclovir should be given (PO 400 mg tds).
- Haze and scarring: The healing response to ablation involves stromal remodelling and restoration of the epithelium. Stromal remodelling involves activation of keratocytes and production of immature collagen matrix which may cause haze through increased light scatter. Mitomycin C applied after ablation reduces this but in doing so may impair the subsequent adhesion of new epithelium through reduced production of junctional adhesion complexes.
- Ectasia: Although only small amounts of tissue are usually removed, if treatments are repeated there is a small risk of weakening the structural integrity of the cornea. This is particularly relevant if the disease process has already affected the biomechanics of the cornea.

2.5 Superficial Keratectomy

2.5.1 Indications

Dense band keratopathy (BKP) and plaque (Fig. 2.19) is sometimes seen affecting eyes with chronic pathology (keratoconjunctivitis sicca, vernal keratoconjunctivitis, uveitis). The lesion may be too dense to be removed with the excimer laser and may require manual removal.

2.5.2 Technique

Under sub-Tenon's block or topical anaesthesia, the epithelium over the keratopathy is brushed back with a hockey stick or crescent blade, which is then used to find the plane between calcification and stroma and elevate an edge. It should then be possible to peel the calcification from the cornea as a thin rigid plaque in one or more pieces. There may be some bleeding from vascularisation. Once all the keratopathy has been removed, a bandage contact lens is placed and the patient is prescribed topical antibiotics (e.g. chloramphenicol qds) and corticosteroids (e.g. dexamethasone qds). Review is in 1 week (Fig. 2.20).

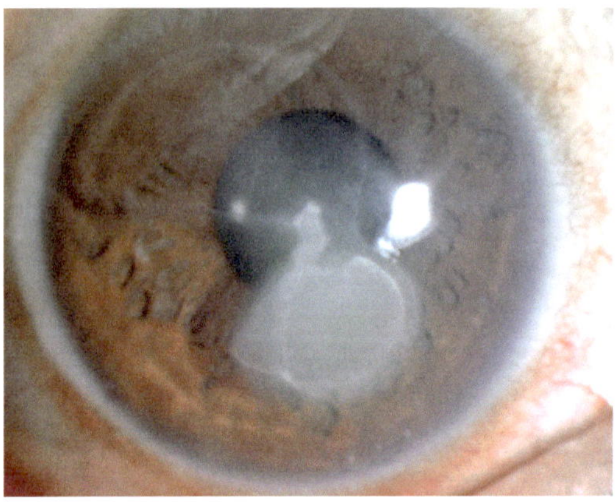

Fig. 2.19 Corneal plaque

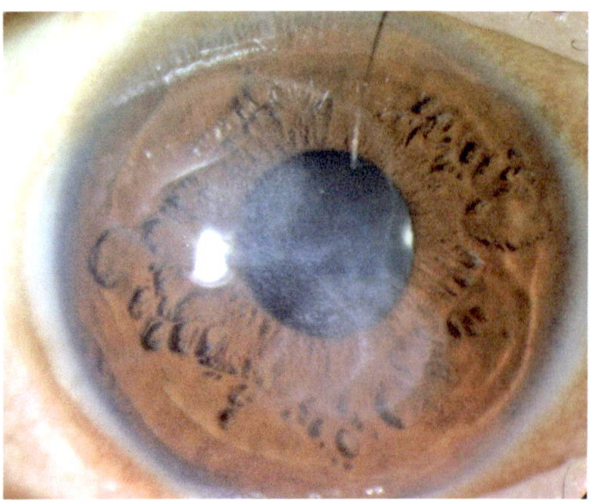

Fig. 2.20 One week after plaque removal (same patient as Fig. 2.19)

2.5.3 Complications

Complications include infection, recurrence, corneal perforation (estimate corneal thickness before starting) and irregular astigmatism.

2.6 Conjunctival Flap

A conjunctival flap can be mobilised over an area of cornea to provide surface protection for a number of reasons. Initially the flap is vascular and opaque but thins and becomes less opaque with time. The cosmetic implications of this should be discussed with the patient before surgery.

2.6.1 Indications and Contraindications

Table 2.3 shows a summary of the indications and contraindications for conjunctival flaps.

2.6.2 Technique

There are two main techniques for conjunctival flaps: Gundersen flap (Fig. 2.21) and pedicle flap.

2.6.2.1 Gundersen Flap

- Used to permanently cover the corneal surface with conjunctiva. The conjunctiva thins and becomes less opaque with time but useful vision is not expected. Cosmesis is usually acceptable and comfort is improved.

Table 2.3 Review plan and treatment after pterygium surgery

Indications	Contraindications
To cover non-healing sterile corneal ulcers or persistent epithelial defects in eyes with limited visual potential	Active infection (although a conjunctival flap can be used for uncontrolled infection, e.g. fungal, in some areas where effective treatment is not available)
Painful bullous keratopathy in eyes with no (or little) useful vision when corneal grafting is not appropriate and conservative measures are unsuccessful	Corneal perforation (unless combined with a corneal graft)
Blind eyes requiring surface protection in preparation for cosmetic prosthetic shell	

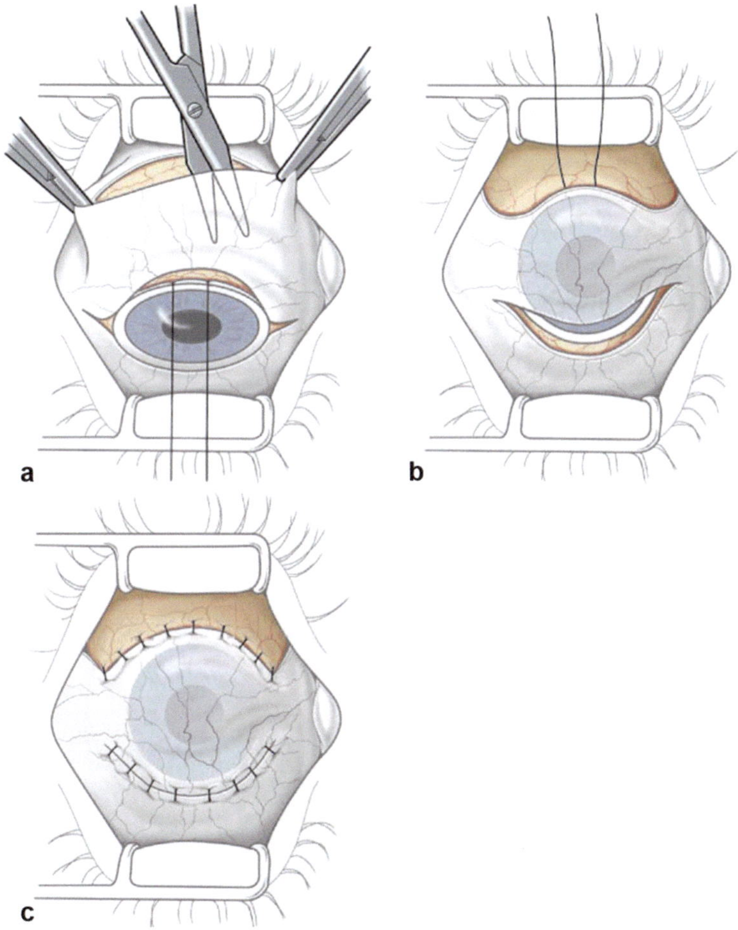

Fig. 2.21 Illustration of Gundersen flap. (**a**) 360° peritomy and superior conjunctival relaxing incision; (**b**) conjunctival flap slides down to cover cornea; (**c**) conjunctival flap secured with 10/0 nylon or vicryl

- Topical, sub-Tenon's or peribulbar anaesthesia is used. Superior bulbar conjunctiva is preferred for the flap, but if conjunctival scarring prevents mobilisation, conjunctiva may be taken from the inferior fornix; the disadvantage of the latter is that less tissue is available.
- A traction suture may be placed in superior peripheral cornea so the eye can be rotated inferiorly to expose superior conjunctiva. Lignocaine 1 % with adrenaline can be used to raise a bleb to start separation of conjunctiva from Tenon's capsule. Dissection with scissors is then used to completely undermine the con-

junctiva and free it from the underlying Tenon layer, paying attention to separate the tissue planes adequately laterally to allow free movement of the conjunctiva without traction. Care must be taken not to buttonhole the conjunctiva. A small buttonhole may be repaired with a purse-string 10/0 vicryl suture. A semicircular incision is made at an appropriate distance posteriorly, parallel to the limbus, and a 360° peritomy is made. Corneal epithelium is removed and the conjunctiva is slid down onto the cornea and secured with 10/0 nylon or vicryl (Fig. 2.22). During formation of a full Gundersen flap, the limbal stem cells are lost. A contact lens can be applied.

- A partial Gundersen flap, for example, for a localised peripheral persistent epithelial defect, can be reversed and a penetrating keratoplasty can be carried out.

2.6.2.2 Pedicle Flap

- To cover a small epithelial defect, perforation or impending perforation (once infection control is established).
- Advantages: The visual axis may be spared, preserving visual function; Tenon's capsule can be taken with the conjunctiva to provide a thicker flap; avascularity of the peripheral cornea is also maintained which is beneficial should a PKP be required later.
- The area of cornea to be covered determines the size of pedicle prepared.

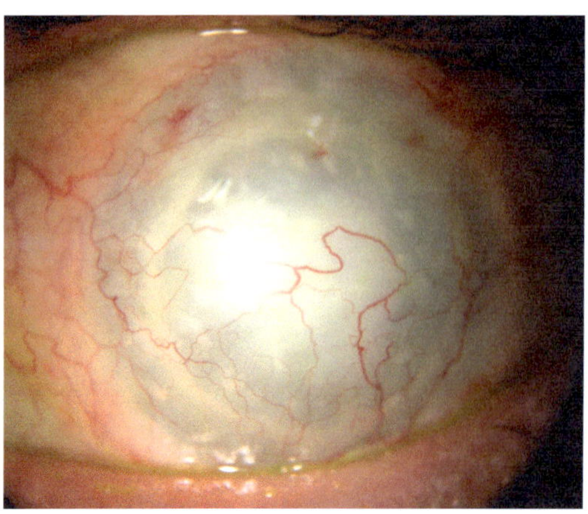

Fig. 2.22 Cornea 6 months after Gundersen conjunctival flap

- A pedicle of conjunctiva is prepared from the upper fornix which is free at one end and ideally contains a prominent blood vessel. Corneal epithelium is scraped from the edge of the defect. The flap is rotated down to cover the epithelial defect and sutured in place with 10/0 nylon. The donor site is closed with 10/0 vicryl. Topical lubricant and broad-spectrum antibiotics are given.

2.7 Amniotic Membrane Transplantation (AMT)

Amniotic membrane (AM) is the inner layer of the foetal membranes, obtained from prospective donors undergoing caesarean section, who are negative for diseases including HIV, hepatitis and syphilis (up to 30 grafts can be prepared from one placenta). The amnion is separated from the chorion by blunt dissection. It has a single epithelial layer, a thick basement membrane and an avascular stroma. It has a number of properties which make it useful in ocular surface restorative surgery: it is sterile, it is non-immunogenic and a good source of growth factors and it has a mild anti-inflammatory and antibacterial effect.

AM is available as fresh tissue or freeze dried and can be prepared with or without its epithelium. Both fresh and preserved AM have been found to function equally well when transplanted onto the ocular surface. The stromal side is shiny and slightly sticky (vitreous-like strands can be raised with a sponge) and is positioned in contact with the target site (epithelial side up). Fresh AM is transported on card with the epithelium up; so it is simply peeled off the card onto the recipient site.

AM does contain living cells but rather facilitates the activity of native limbal stem cells. AMT alone is therefore not sufficient in cases of severe limbal ischaemia or total stem cell failure.

By law, serologic tests on the maternal donor must be done both at the time of procurement of the donor tissue and again 6 months later. This dual testing minimises risk of disease transmission.

2.7.1 Indication

- To facilitate epithelialisation in cases of mild limbal stem cell deficiency (Fig. 2.23) or persistent epithelial defect
- To facilitate epithelialisation and reduce scarring after chemical injuries (especially alkali injuries)
- To reduce pain and aid re-epithelialisation after corneal surgery, particularly superficial keratectomy or recurrent pterygia

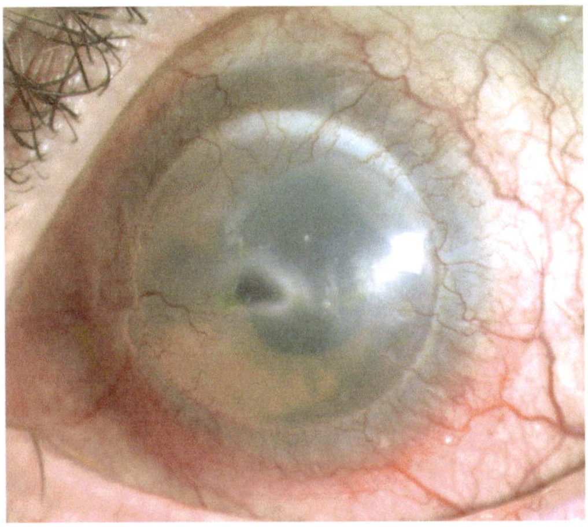

Fig. 2.23 Corneal vascularisation in stem cell deficiency

2.7.2 Technique

AM can be used as a substrate for epithelium to grow on top of (inlay technique) or as a physiological dressing for epithelium to grow underneath (overlay technique). The techniques are illustrated in Fig. 2.24.

2.7.2.1 Inlay Technique (Graft Technique)

The inlay technique is indicated for areas of stromal loss, for example, melting or deep ulcers. Loose epithelium is debrided. The edge of the area to be covered is undermined slightly at the base with a crescent blade and the AM sized to overlap the defect by 1–2 mm. The edge of AM is then tucked into the undermined edge and secured with 10/0 vicryl. The suture pass is directed firstly through the AM, then into the undermined groove and out through the corneal surface. When tied, the suture should be rotated in the same direction to tension the AM into the groove rather than dragging it back out. The tension must be such that the graft is held snugly and evenly in the base of the defect without the sutures being so tight that they tear out. A bandage contact lens is placed and topical antibiotic and lubricant eye drops are given. In this situation

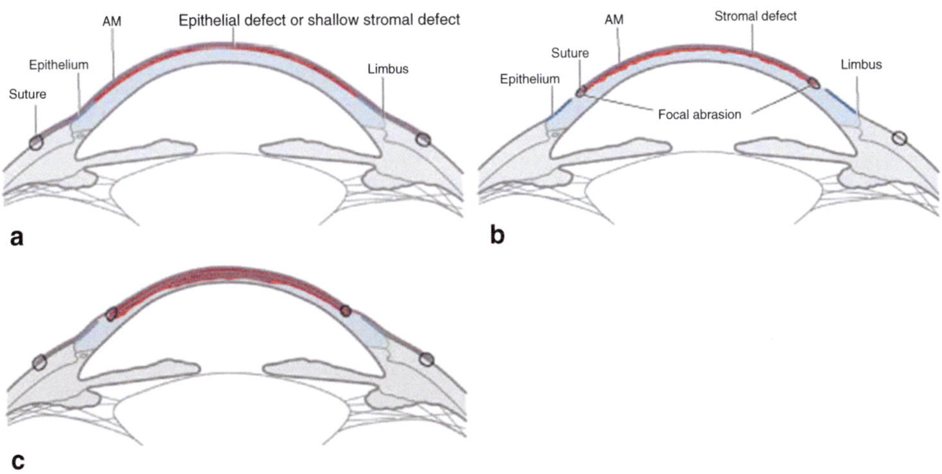

Fig. 2.24 Illustration of amniotic membrane transplantation (AMT). (**a**) Overlay technique covering cornea and limbus: AMT acts as a biological protective covering; (**b**) inlay technique: AMT used as a substrate to facilitate corneal re-epithelialisation; (**c**) deep stromal defect filled in with multiple layers of AMT (sutured in place) and covered with onlay AMT

the AM is covered by the new epithelium causing reduced corneal transparency for some months until it is absorbed.

2.7.2.2 Overlay Technique (Patch Technique)

This is effectively a biological contact lens. The area of cornea and/or conjunctiva to be covered is identified and sufficient AM is used to cover the area completely. More than one piece may be needed. The AM is slid onto the recipient cornea and secured around the limbus with a combination of interrupted and continuous 10/0 vicryl. Suture bites must secure the AM into the episclera rather than just fixing it to the conjunctiva. If large areas of conjunctiva are affected, for example, after a chemical injury, AM may be sutured into the fornices to prevent symblepharon. Double-ended 6/0 polypropylene sutures are used to anchor AM deep into the fornix and brought out through the lid skin, secured over bolsters. The edge of the palpebral piece of AM is secured to the lash line with continuous 10/0 nylon. A bandage contact lens is placed and topical antibiotic and lubricant drops are given. Since the AM is not transparent, the vision is obscured somewhat, but as the epithelium underneath heals, the AM sloughs off at around 10–14 days, at which point the nylon sutures are removed. Some surgeons apply multiple layers of AM.

2.7.2.3 Filling-In Technique

In this technique the depth of a deep corneal ulcer is filled with trimmed, small pieces of AM (multilayered approach) and finally covered with AM (overlay technique).

2.8 Tarsorrhaphy

Physically closing or part closing the eyelids provides protection to the ocular surface and may help an epithelial defect (neurotrophic keratitis) to heal. It is also used to prevent exposure keratopathy in cases where prolonged lagophthalmos is expected, for example, following surgical trauma to the facial nerve.

2.8.1 Temporary Tarsorrhaphy

A temporary tarsorrhaphy is usually placed to close the lateral aspect of the palpebral aperture (Fig. 2.25) but can be placed centrally or medially (or a combination, Fig. 2.26) as required. A temporary tarsorrhaphy beforehand may help determine whether a permanent tarsorrhaphy will be beneficial and will help the patient to adjust cosmetically and functionally.

2.8.1.1 Technique

- The eyelids are infiltrated with 1 or 2 % lignocaine with adrenaline. Bolsters are cut from the silicone tube of a butterfly phlebotomy set, 3–4 mm in length.
- A double-ended 4/0 or 5/0 polypropylene suture is used. The needle is passed through upper lid skin at the superior edge of the temporal third of the tarsal plate, down through the tarsal plate and out through the grey line. This

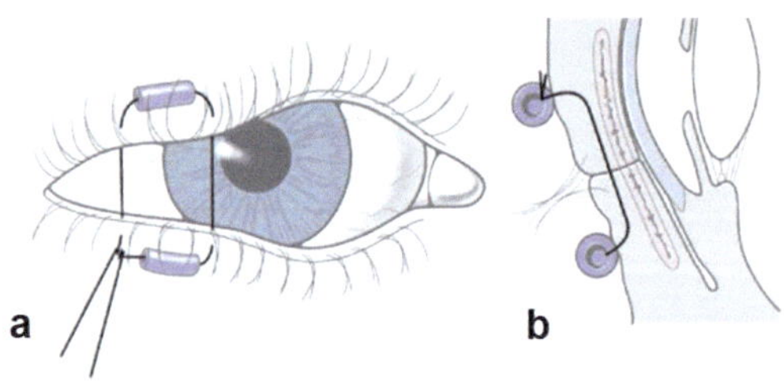

Fig. 2.25 Illustration of temporal temporary tarsorrhaphy. (**a**) Lateral temporary tarsorrhaphy before tightening sutures; (**b**) saggital view of eyelids with tarsorrhaphy in situ

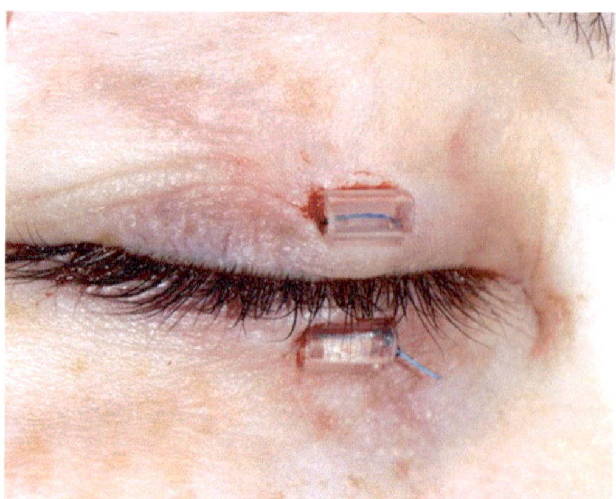

Fig. 2.26 Temporary tarsorrhaphy (early postoperative; photo courtesy of Brian Leatherbarrow)

path is followed in reverse for the lower lid (i.e. grey line-tarsal plate-out through skin). The other needle is threaded through a 3–4 mm length of bolster tubing and then passes through the lids parallel to the first, approx 5 mm away. Care must be taken not to damage the globe.

- Passage of the sutures through tarsus is essential for tensile strength; if the suture passes just through skin, there is a high chance that it will cut out.
- The two needles are passed through a second silicone bolster and tied so that their ends do not poke into lid skin or risk abrading the cornea.
- Tension in the sutures should hold the lid margins firmly together.
- A second double-ended suture tied over bolsters can be placed next to the first for additional lid closure.
- A small palpebral opening should be left medially to allow instillation of drops and examination of the cornea (a slip knot can be used to allow corneal inspection).

2.8.2 Permanent Tarsorrhaphy

A permanent tarsorrhaphy is considered for cases when long-term protection is needed, for example, when return of lid closure function is not anticipated.

2.8.2.1 Technique

- The eyelids are infiltrated with 1 or 2 % lignocaine with adrenaline.
- The anterior and posterior lid lamellae are split (upper and lower).
- Using a no. 15 blade, a strip of the lid margin is excised from the posterior lamellae where the permanent closure is required. The lash line should be spared.
- The exposed edges of tarsal plates are sutured together with 6/0 vicryl, keeping the knot away from the ocular surface.
- The anterior lamellae are sutured together with 6/0 prolene over bolsters.
- Chloramphenicol ointment is given at the end of the procedure qds for 1 week, then lubricants as appropriate. Once the edges have healed together (usually 2 weeks), the bolsters can be removed.
- For a more secure closure, a 'tongue' of upper lid tarsus can be freed at one end and sutured down into a corresponding groove removed from the lower lid tarsus. This is harder to reverse.

2.8.3 Tarsorrhaphy Removal

Reversal of a permanent tarsorrhaphy is possible, but care must be taken not to damage the globe under the apposed lids. After infiltration with local anaesthetic, a small malleable retractor can be placed between the surface of the eye and the lids to give protection while the lids are separated with scissors or a no. 15 blade. Once separated, careful pinpoint cautery can be used for haemostasis. The patient should be counselled regarding the chance of lid margin asymmetry and possible need to replace the tarsorrhaphy.

2.8.4 Alternative Treatment Options

2.8.4.1 Gluing

In cases where it is preferable to avoid any surgery (very elderly or uncontrolled anticoagulant status), a temporary tarsorrhaphy can be achieved by gluing the upper lashes down onto the lower lid skin with cyanoacrylate glue. Care must be taken not to introduce glue onto the ocular surface or into the fornices as it will cause trauma as it hardens. Spontaneous separation is observed in around 7–10 days.

2.8.4.2 Botulinum Toxin Injection

Injection of botulinum toxin A to the levator palpebrae superioris (5–10 units of Botox™) results in lid closure while permitting full access to the cornea for examination. Onset occurs around 5 days after injection and the effect lasts for 8–12 weeks. Injection should be through the upper eyelid above the skin crease just into the pre-aponeurotic fat pad. Complications of injection include globe perforation and diplopia due to hypotropia persisting after ptosis resolves. The use of botulinum toxin is contraindicated in neuromuscular diseases such as myasthenia gravis.

2.9 Lacrimal Occlusion

Occlusion of the lacrimal puncta can potentiate tears or topical medications and aid healing. Occlusion can be temporary or permanent. Lower (70 % of the normal drainage), upper or both puncta can be occluded depending on how much reduction in tear drainage is required.

2.9.1 Temporary Lacrimal Occlusion

Various types of punctal plugs are available:

- Cellulose cylinders which are inserted into the canaliculus are well tolerated but tend to fall out. It can be difficult to tell later whether the device is still in situ or has become displaced.
- Silicone plugs which are shaped to sit at the punctum with a flange to prevent movement in or out. These come in various sizes (0.4–0.8 mm) so the sizing instrument can be used to help decide which size to select; the plug should fit in tightly. The patient is sometimes aware of a foreign body sensation, and if not inserted correctly, the plug may abrade the cornea or can cause a granuloma. Removal at the slit lamp is quick and easy using a fine non-toothed forceps.

2.9.2 Permanent Lacrimal Occlusion

Cautery of the punctum achieves permanent occlusion and should only be done after a trial of temporary occlusion to ensure that this is well tolerated and does not cause intolerable epiphora. Technique: local anaesthetic is infiltrated under the eyelid skin by the punctum. Under the operating microscope a fine cautery instrument is inserted into the punctum and the tissues cauterised to induce closure (by scarring).

2.10 Stem Cell Transplantation

Stem cells are immature cells that have the potential to become specialised into different types of cells throughout the body. Adult stem cells (also found in children) are stem cells that reside in already developed tissue, acting like a repair system and providing new specialised cells to take the place of those that are lost.

Corneal epithelial stem cells have been demonstrated to reside in the limbal epithelium, while the fornical zone of the conjunctiva appears to be a predominant site of conjunctival epithelial stem cells. However, specific identification of cell markers of limbal stem cells has proved elusive. Conjunctivalisation and vascularisation of the corneal surface and persistent or recurring epithelial defects are hallmarks of limbal stem cell deficiency.

Limbal stem cell deficiency is one of the many causes of a loss in corneal transparency. In cases of an ocular surface failure following chemical burn involving the limbus, the only effective management is a stem cell transplant. Other indications for a limbal stem cell transplant include ocular surface disease and trauma, ocular pemphigoid and Stevens-Johnson syndrome.

For unilateral disease to perform a stem cell transplant, the surgeon takes limbal stem cells from the patient's healthy fellow eye (autograft) or from the healthy eye of a living relative or cadaver (allograft) if there is bilateral disease (Fig. 2.27).

After the transplantation patients are treated with topical antibiotics, topical corticosteroids and oral corticosteroids. Oral immunosuppressives are required with allografts.

2.11 Corneal Cross-Linking

Corneal collagen cross-linking (CXL) enhances the stiffness of the cornea. The principle is that extra cross links are created between bundles of collagen fibres, increasing tissue stiffness. It has been used to stabilise the cornea in keratoconus,

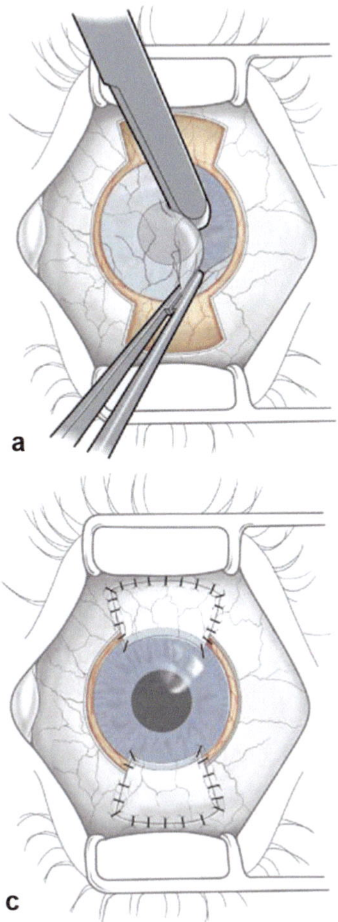

Fig. 2.27 Illustration of stem cell transplantation (SCT). (**a**) Removing corneal pannus (recipient eye); (**b**) taking donor stem cell niche (donor eye); (**c**) donor material secured to recipient eye

pellucid marginal degeneration and bullous keratopathy. It has also been evaluated as an adjunct to treat infection and corneal melting. The aim is to prevent progression of the disease process, and an improvement in visual acuity is sometimes seen.

The technique relies upon the combination of a photosensitising substance (riboflavin) and UVA light to increase the number of covalent bonds between and within collagen fibrils. It also increases collagen resistance to enzymatic destruction.

Riboflavin eye drops are applied to the de-epithelialised (or epithelialised) cornea. When the riboflavin has penetrated sufficiently, the cornea is illuminated by UVA light to activate the riboflavin which induces cross links. Riboflavin saturation in the corneal stroma induces free-radical formation and also acts as a shield to protect deeper structures (e.g. damage to the endothelium) by absorbing the ultraviolet energy.

2.11.1 Indications and Contraindications

Indications include:

- Conditions where corneal structural integrity is compromised with documented evidence of progression of ectasia (keratoconus, refractive surgery).
- Strengthening of superficial laminae and reduction of bulla formation in bullous keratopathy.
- CXL has also been successfully used to treat antimicrobial-resistant infectious keratitis since the procedure also kills bacteria and fungi.

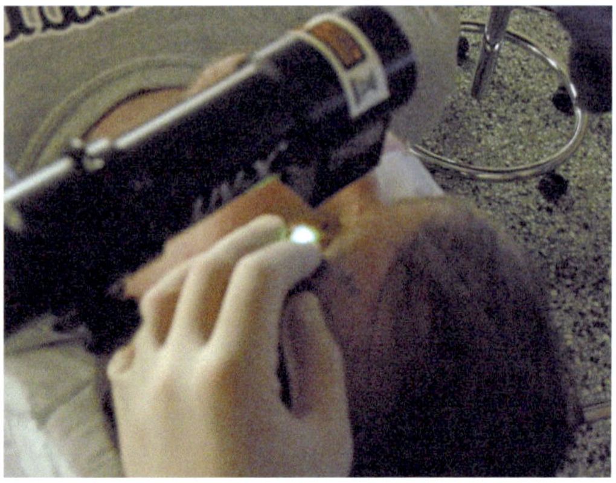

Fig. 2.28 Corneal cross-linking

Contraindications include history of herpetic keratitis, pregnancy, active infection and autoimmune disease.

2.11.2 Technique

Topical anaesthetic is applied and the epithelium is removed. Riboflavin 0.1 % eye drops in dextran 20 % solution are given every 3 min for 15 min to ensure adequate corneal penetration. This can be judged at the slit lamp by observing riboflavin in the anterior chamber. UVA irradiation at 3 mW/cm^2 is applied for 30 min during which time further riboflavin drops are given every 2 min (Fig. 2.28). A bandage contact lens is applied and the patient is prescribed topical antibiotic and lubricant drops. The contact lens is removed at 1 month and the drops tapered over 6 weeks.

CXL can be performed without removing the epithelium but this is less effective. Topical anaesthetic or other agent (e.g. benzalkonium chloride) is used to compromise the tight junctions between epithelial cells which usually provide a barrier against penetration. Weakening the epithelial barrier in this way allows riboflavin to penetrate, but this is less efficient.

The KXL System (Avedro) allows for accelerated corneal cross-linking. By increasing the UVA power (30 mW/cm^2) and reducing the exposure time (3 min), the cross-linking time can be reduced, but the same energy on the eye (5.4 J/ cm^2) can be maintained.

Key points for the assessment:

- Preoperative thickness of the de-epithelialised central cornea must exceed 400 μm.
- The patient must be counselled regarding the unpredictability of the treatment and the possible need for further surgery, for example, intracorneal ring segments or keratoplasty.

2.11.3 Complications

Complications include failure, corneal melt, infection and scarring.

3 Corneal Transplantation

3.1 Indications and Techniques

In the UK approximately 3,000 and in the USA approximately 45,000 corneal transplants are carried out each year. The main indications for corneal transplantation are listed in Table 3.1. The most common indications are corneal ectasia (Figs. 3.1, 3.2 and 3.3), corneal dystrophy (Figs. 3.4 and 3.5), corneal scarring and vascularisation (Figs. 3.6 and 3.7), corneal decompensation (Fig. 3.8) and corneal perforation (Fig. 3.9).

Evolution of surgical techniques over the last two decades has allowed a shift from penetrating keratoplasty being the procedure of choice in all cases to lamellar keratoplasty for selective replacement of the diseased tissue with preservation of healthy host tissue where possible (Fig. 3.10). This improves structural integrity and potentially reduces the risks of rejection.

In 1999, 86 % of corneal transplants were penetrating keratoplasties, but by 2009 this had dropped to only 55 % of grafts. Over this time the rate of lamellar grafts rose from only 4 % in 1999 (all deep anterior) to over a third in 2009 when 11 % of corneal grafts were deep anterior lamellar keratoplasties and 23 % were endothelial replacement procedures. The remaining transplant procedures were limbal stem cell transplants or corneo-scleral procedures.

For disorders of anterior lamellae (i.e. epithelium and stroma), a deep anterior lamellar keratoplasty (DALK) can be considered. For disorders of Descemet's membrane or endothelium, a selective replacement of Descemet's and endothelium can be considered, such as Descemet's stripping endothelial keratoplasty (DSEK), Descemet's stripping automated endothelial keratoplasty (DSAEK) or Descemet's membrane endothelial keratoplasty (DMEK). For disorders of peripheral cornea or corneo-scleral melts, a crescentic corneal or corneo-scleral graft may be the most suitable option. For patients with limbal stem cell deficiency, a limbal stem cell transplant can be offered, either as an autograft from the fellow eye if there is sufficient healthy limbal stem cells (LSC) remaining or an allograft if not. For conditions affecting all corneal layers, penetrating keratoplasty remains an excellent option.

3.2 Patient Consent

Corneal transplant surgery is only one part of the process, and the long visual rehabilitation period requires a strong and stable doctor-patient relationship. A patient's motivation to comply with treatment and attend for follow-up for up to 2 years is as much a key to a successful outcome as technical excellence in the operating theatre.

It is vital that the patient understands the nature of the surgery and the risks and potential complications involved. Time should be spent at the earliest practical opportunity to discuss the implications of embarking on this journey and to allow the patient to consider their options and ask questions. Written information booklets should be available for patients to keep and read in their own time.

The patient must have realistic expectation. The earlier this is assessed, the more likely it is

B. Zuberbuhler et al., *Corneal Surgery*,
DOI 10.1007/978-3-642-12502-7_3,

Table 3.1 Indications for corneal transplantation

Optical > improve vision	Therapeutic > relieve pain	Tectonic > restore structure	Cosmetic > restore appearance
74 %	20 %	3 %	3 %[a]
Keratoconus Corneal scars Pseudophakic bullous keratopathy Fuchs' endothelial dystrophy Graft failure High refractive error	Bullous keratopathy	Corneal perforation Corneal melt	Congenital opacities

[a]Australian graft registry 1997

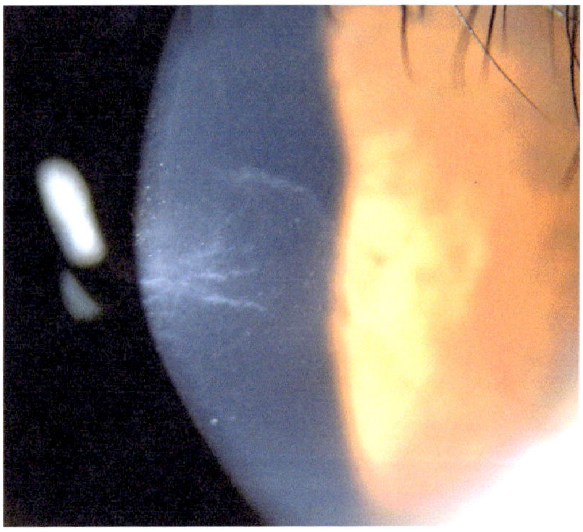

Fig. 3.1 Keratoconus with Vogt striae

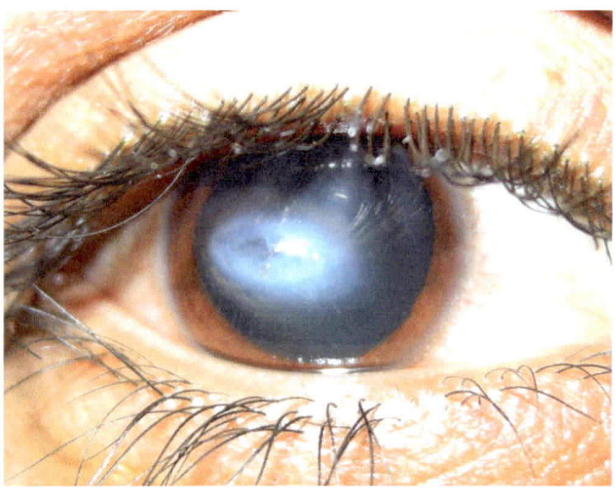

Fig. 3.2 Corneal hydrops in keratoconus

that unrealistic expectations can be modified. Patients may benefit from discussion with specialist nurses or with other patients who have had surgery for similar conditions so that they are more able to imagine how the transplant will affect them and what level of visual performance can be realistically anticipated.

Informed consent for surgery should be documented after a discussion between patient and surgeon which covers at least the following:

- Type of surgery planned and other procedures which may be necessary
- Indication for surgery
- Risks including graft failure (primary or delayed), rejection, infection, raised intraocular pressure (development or worsening of glaucoma), cataract, suture-related problems (loose/broken suture, suture infection) and loss of vision and possible need for further procedures including suture adjustment, suture removal, graft re-suturing, regrafting, arcuate keratotomies, phakic IOL, LASIK, LASEK or PRK
- Type of anaesthetic planned

A copy of the signed consent form should be given to the patient to keep.

3.3 Specific Equipment

3.3.1 Ophthalmic Viscoelastic Devices

Ophthalmic viscoelastic devices (OVDs) are used in all types of corneal grafting to protect the endothelium, to create or maintain space in the eye. OVD should be completely aspirated at the end of surgery.

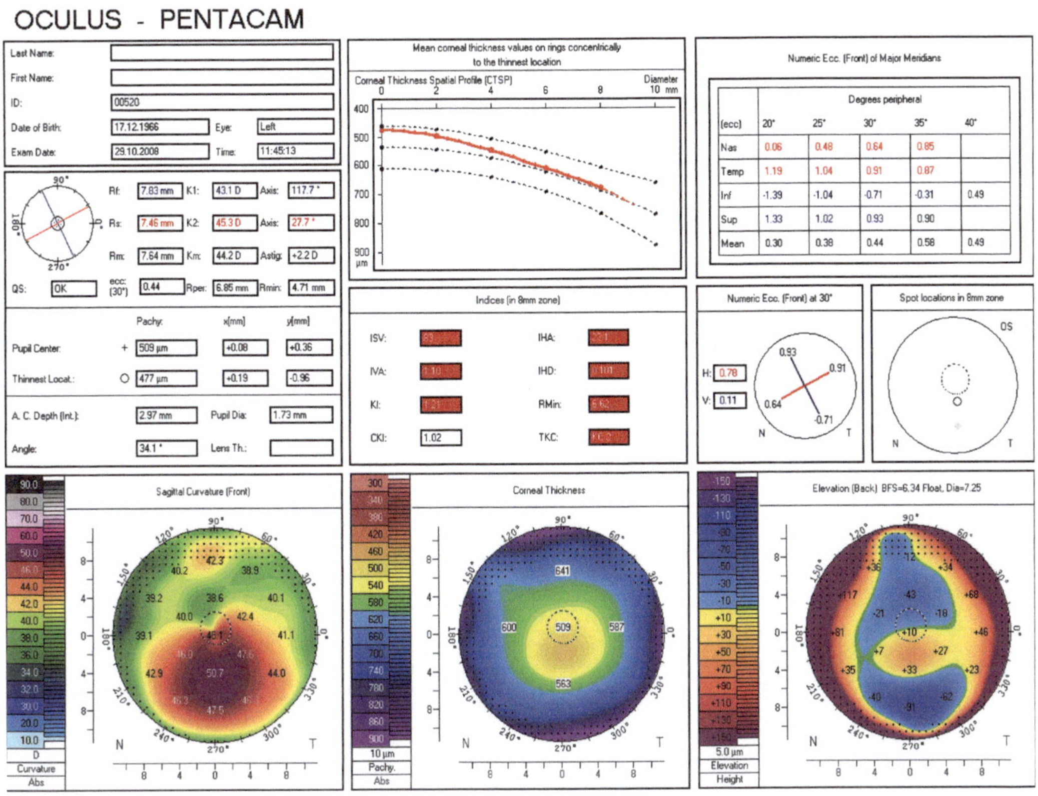

Fig. 3.3 Printout Pentacam Keratoconus Grade 2

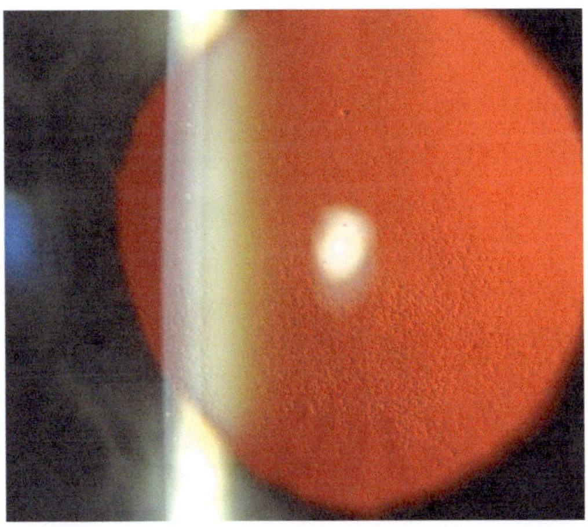

Fig. 3.4 Fuchs' endothelial dystrophy

3.3.1.1 Penetrating Keratoplasty

During penetrating keratoplasty once the trephine has penetrated into the anterior chamber, the release of aqueous tends to allow the anterior chamber to collapse. A cohesive OVD of medium viscosity (e.g. Healon, ProVisc) may be used to reform the anterior chamber so that the excision can be completed with scissors or a blade. OVD is added to the 'open eye' once the host tissue is removed to form a bed onto which the donor can be safely placed.

3.3.1.2 Deep Anterior Lamellar Keratoplasty

During Melles' technique for deep anterior lamellar keratoplasty, once the lamellar dissection is complete the pre-Descemet's membrane space is opened by injecting OVD into the dissection plane so that Descemet's membrane is kept away from the trephine used to remove the host stroma. The use of OVD is also essential when performing 'big-bubble' deep anterior lamellar keratoplasty.

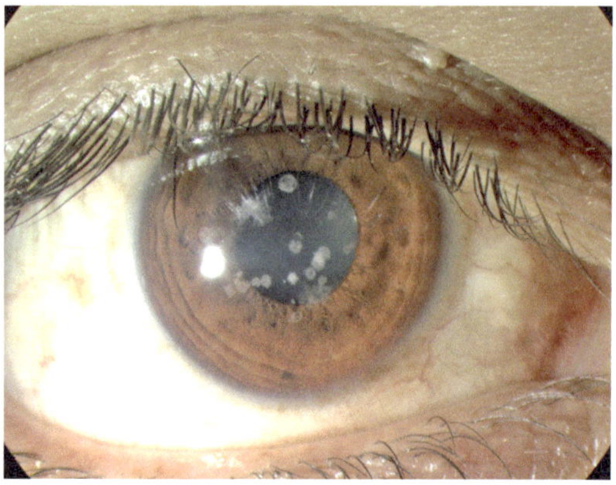

Fig. 3.5 Moderate granular corneal dystrophy, asymptomatic

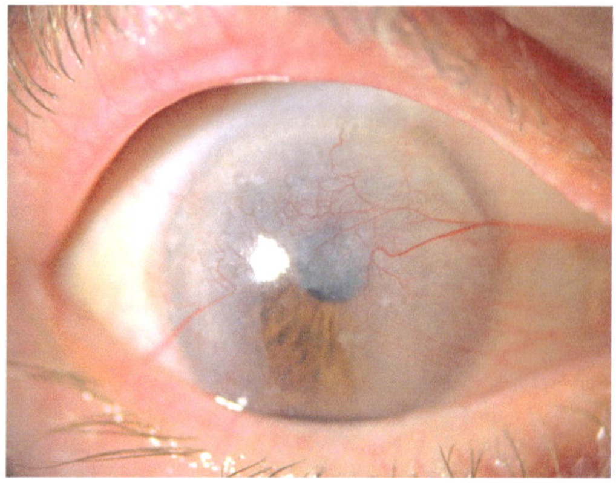

Fig. 3.7 Corneal vascularisation in Stevens-Johnsons syndrome (or ocular rosacea)

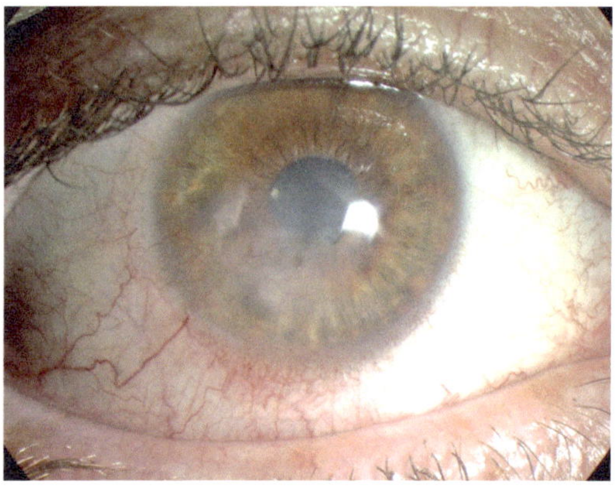

Fig. 3.6 Corneal scar from recurrent herpes simplex keratitis

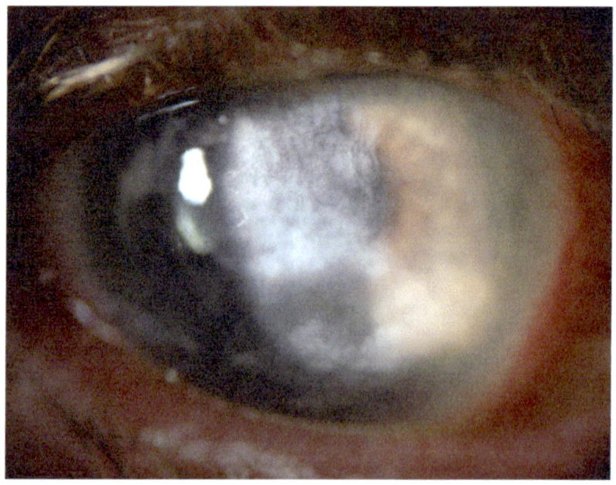

Fig. 3.8 Corneal decompensation with scarring

3.3.1.3 Descemet's Stripping Endothelial Keratoplasty

During Descemet's stripping endothelial keratoplasty, a cohesive OVD is used to maintain the AC, while DM and endothelium are stripped but must be removed before the graft is introduced. Dispersive OVDs must be avoided since complete removal is harder to guarantee and any OVD remaining at the graft-host interface will impair graft adhesion. A small amount of OVD is also used to protect the endothelium from trauma while it is introduced into the eye.

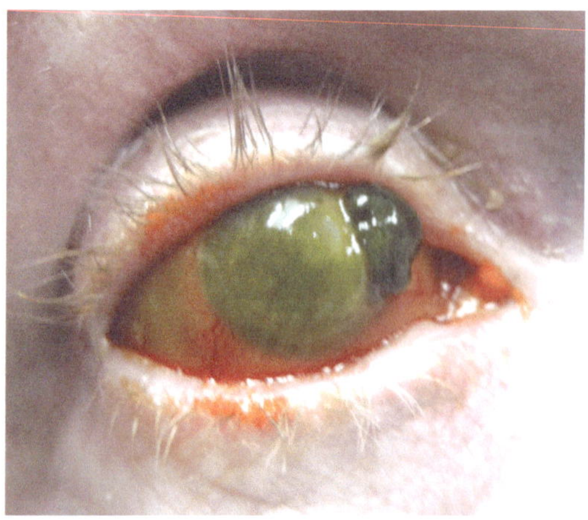

Fig. 3.9 Corneal melt with iris prolapsed

3.3.2 Scleral Rings

Scleral rings are support devices sutured to the sclera to give added support to the eye and prevent scleral collapse during penetrating keratoplasty. This is indicated if the eye's inherent support is weak, for example, aphakic or vitrectomised eyes, or in children in whom the

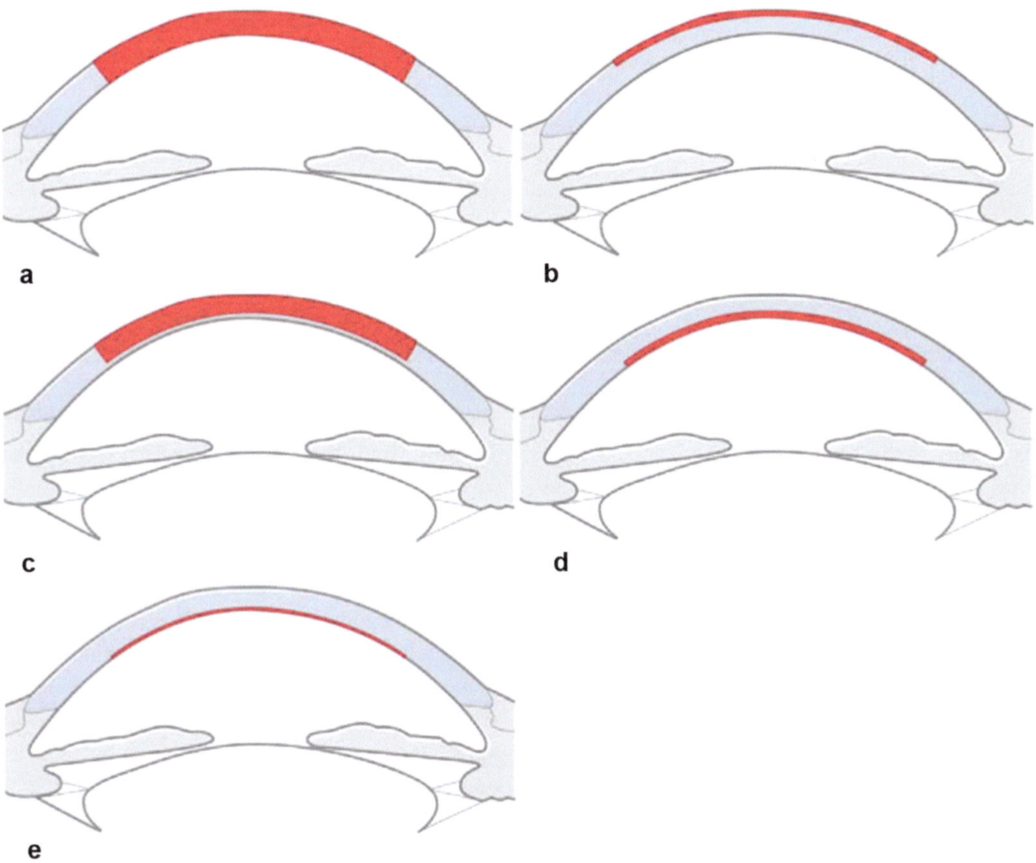

Fig. 3.10 Illustration of keratoplasty techniques (penetrating, anterior and posterior lamellar). (**a**) Penetrating keratoplasty; (**b**) superficial anterior lamellar keratoplasty; (**c**) deep anterior lamellar keratoplasty; (**d**) Descemet stripping endothelial keratoplasty; (**e**) Descemet's membrane endothelial keratoplasty

sclera is not sufficiently rigid to maintain adequate tissue support.

Various types and sizes are available, for example, Flieringa rings (15–19 mm). The ring is sutured to the sclera with 7/0 vicryl using four radially oriented sutures before trephining the cornea. Care must be taken to ensure even tension around the circumference to avoid inducing astigmatism. Care must also be taken to avoid full-thickness suture bites which would risk causing a retinal hole or bleeding from the ciliary body. The ring is removed at the end of the operation.

3.3.3 Corneal Trephines

Zirm's first successful human corneal transplant in 1905 used the von Hippel trephine. Designed in 1886, this had a circular cutting edge on a long shaft which was rotated by a wind-up mechanism. Advances in technology and materials have allowed the evolution of trephines towards the devices we are familiar with today. Modern trephines allow host and donor tissue to be cut with precision in terms of size and shape to reduce induced astigmatism. Principally, suction trephines consist of an outer circular chamber of small volume connected to a spring-loaded syringe and an inner circular blade advanced by rotating along a screw thread.

3.3.3.1 Sizing

Trephines are available in many different sizes, often in sizes from 6.0 to 7.0 mm in 0.5 mm steps and from 7.0 to 9.0 mm in 0.25 mm steps. For most eyes, the optimal size is between 7.5 and 8 mm. Donor corneas that are too small may cause higher astigmatism and the sutures may interfere with the visual axis, while corneas that

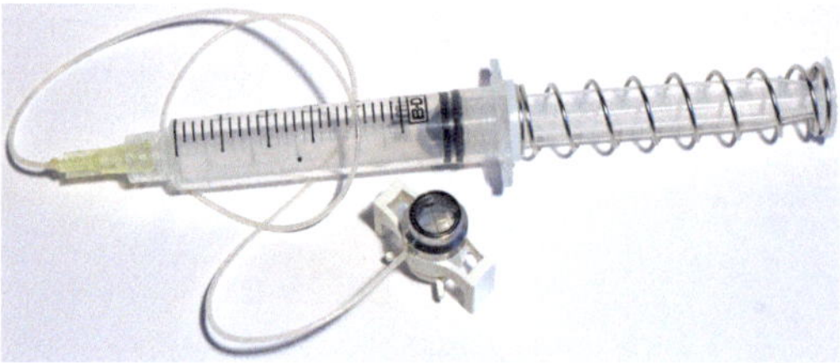

Fig. 3.11 Barron radial vacuum trephine (Katena)

are too large bear higher risks of vascularisation, rejection, glaucoma and iris incarceration.

Cut from the endothelial site, the donor button is usually 0.25–0.5 mm larger ('oversized') than that excised from the host to aid healing and wound apposition, and also to compensate for the profile created in the host rim if a suction trephine is used. Oversized donors have more endothelial cells and are therefore beneficial for Fuchs' endothelial dystrophy and pseudophakic bullous keratopathy. Oversizing should not be done for patients younger than 50 years. Same-size donor corneas may be used for keratoconus (optimal 8 mm diameter) and high myopes (more than 6 D (dioptres)).

Other approaches to decide on the size of the donor have been presented, for example, same size for eyes up to 7 mm donor diameter, minimal oversize (+0.25 mm) for donor corneas between 7 and 8.5 mm and moderate oversize (+0.5 mm) for donor corneas of more than 8.5 mm diameter.

3.3.3.2 Disposable Suction Trephines (Type)

Disposable trephines, for example, Barron radial vacuum trephine, Katena (Fig. 3.11), are a preferred choice as a sharp edge can be guaranteed without the risk of cutting edges becoming irregular due to imperfect resharpening as was encountered in the era of reusable trephines.

The blade must be checked under the microscope for irregularities before use, advanced until it is flush with the suction ring and then withdrawn slightly. The blade has cross hairs which indicate the centre of rotation and aid alignment to the centre of the cornea, which has been marked with a marker pen. The plunger of the syringe is depressed, the trephine is placed onto the centre of the cornea and the syringe released to create a vacuum which holds the trephine firmly in place. Creation of the vacuum is a crucial step as loss of suction during cutting may lead to significant irregularity in the cut. The inner blade is then rotated; it advances 250 μm for each 360° rotation.

3.3.3.3 Handheld Trephines

Handheld trephines are similar to those used for dermatological punch biopsies. The circular blade may be mounted on a plastic handle or held between the finger and thumb and rotated to trephine the cornea. Gentle pressure is applied as a partial-thickness cut is made. This can then be safely extended to full thickness with a diamond blade without risking an uncontrolled full-thickness trephination and anterior chamber collapse.

Handheld trephines are an alternative to suction trephines when performing a tectonic graft for a patient with a corneal perforation to reduce the risk of expulsion of globe contents as suction is applied. However, they tend to result in more astigmatism than suction trephines as they are prone to tilt or create an eccentric cut. Unexpected anterior chamber entry is also a possibility and trephine with long handles may be difficult to use under the microscope. Trephines are available in stepped sizes from 4.0 to 14.0 mm (Medtronic Ophthalmics; 1.0, 0.5 or 0.25 mm steps variously).

3.3.3.4 Motorised Trephines

The Asmotom (Deutschmann Instruments, Germany) vacuum fixates both the peripheral cornea and the central corneal button and uses a motorised blade to cut to a preset depth. Donor buttons of 6.0, 6.5, 7.1, 7.6 and 8.2 mm can be prepared. The recipient cornea can be cut to 6.0, 6.5, 7.0, 7.5 and 8.0 mm.

3.3.3.5 Femtosecond Laser

The femtosecond laser is an alternative to traditional blade-based systems and is becoming more widespread in its applications in corneal surgery. It uses focussed laser energy at infrared wavelengths to separate intermolecular bonds in tissues. The

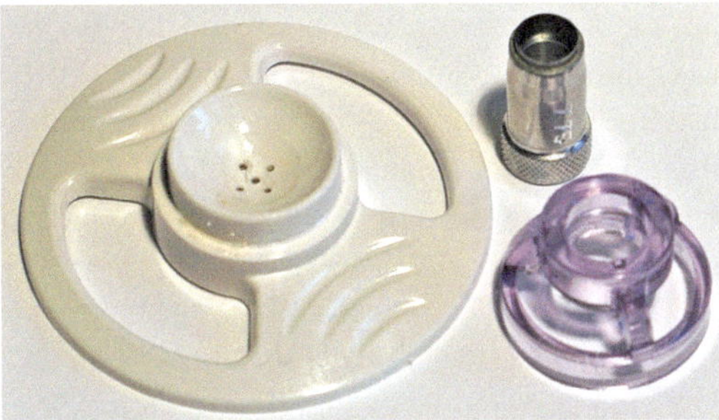

Fig. 3.12 Coronet donor punch set (Angiotech)

energy can be focussed precisely enabling cuts to be made in tissue to very precise depths and patterns. This allows surgeons to match host and donor tissue more closely than ever before and to be creative in planning the profile of keratoplasty incisions. For example, a 'top-hat' profile allows transplantation of a greater area of endothelium without the anterior portion of the graft-host interface being too close to the limbus and increasing the risk of rejection. A zigzag configuration creates a larger area of graft-host adherence, increasing the mechanical strength of the interface and reducing the risk of globe rupture. The main disadvantages of this are the instrument cost, limited availability, the extra time required and the lack of evidence of clinical superiority.

3.3.4 Cutting Blocks

The process of obtaining the donor button has likewise evolved over time. The most common method currently is to place the donor corneoscleral disc endothelium-up on a concave block, centering it carefully, for example, Coronet donor punch set, Angiotech (Fig. 3.12). The periphery of the block has holes in it to accommodate pegs on the cutter's base to ensure alignment. The cutter is fitted and pressed down firmly to cut a full-thickness donor button. Corneas punched from the endothelium side are often smaller than attempted (about 0.2 mm less) which is taken into account when sizing (usually 0.25 oversized).

Variations on this theme exist which use spring-loaded or dropped-weight arrangements to create the cutting force. To minimise any movement of the donor tissue before cutting, vacuum can be applied through holes in the base of the block from a spring-loaded syringe (as per suction trephine).

Some cutting instruments allow cutting the corneal tissue from the epithelial side. The corneo-scleral disc is placed on an anterior chamber maintainer and the device pressurised with saline or viscoelastic. A suction trephine is then used to cut the donor button. The main benefit of this is that host and graft profiles should match more closely, but the procedure is more time consuming and the equipment is more expensive.

3.3.5 Anterior Lamellar Dissection

Superficial anterior lamellar keratoplasty (SALK) can be carried out with a microkeratome similar to that used for LASIK procedures. The blade depth is typically set around 140–160 μm. The Amadeus microkeratome (Schwind) can be used to prepare donor tissue with the Mozart artificial anterior chamber and the recipient cornea. This system also allows lamellae up to 250 μm thick for SALK. An 8.5 mm suction ring is used, and the blade is changed between donor and recipient cutting.

3.3.6 Posterior Lamellar Dissection

The thin posterior lamellar graft required for endothelial keratoplasty can be prepared manually by lamellar dissection (for DSEK) or by a microkeratome (for DSAEK). The microkeratomes currently available for this are the Moria ALTK, the Med-Logics ML7 and the Schwind system. The donor cornea is usually prepared by the surgeon in theatre, but some eye banks (particularly in the USA) are now supplying pre-cut lamellar grafts. It is likely that this will also become more widely available in other countries in the near future.

The Moria LSK/ALTK/CBm microkeratome (Figs. 3.13 and 3.14) combines an artificial anterior chamber with a microkeratome. The depth of cut can be set at 300 μm for corneas of thickness <570 or 350 μm for corneas of thickness ≥570 μm. The donor corneo-scleral disc must be between 16 and 19 mm diameter. The artificial anterior chamber (Fig. 3.15) holds the donor cornea securely with viscoelastic protecting the endothelium, while the microkeratome removes an anterior cap of stroma leaving behind the graft consisting of endothelium, DM and a thin layer of stroma. The lamellar graft is transferred to a block and punched from the endothelial side.

The Schwind artificial anterior chamber is a similar device which is compatible with the Schwind Carriazo-Pendular microkeratome. This system can be used for anterior lamellar grafts as well as DSAEK and has four ring sizes between 8.5 and 10 mm and cutting heads for depths of 300, 350 or 400 μm.

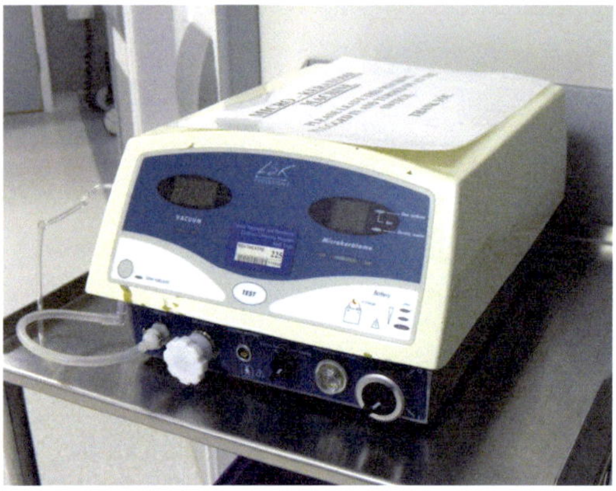

Fig. 3.13 Moria SLK Evolution 2 Control Unit

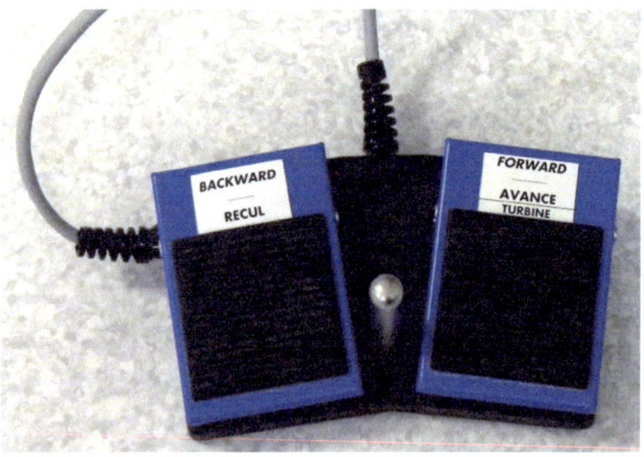

Fig. 3.14 Moria SLK Evolution 2 Pedals

3.3.7 Artificial Anterior Chamber

The artificial anterior chamber (AC), for example, Barron artificial anterior chamber, Katena (Fig. 3.16), is a device on which a donor cornea is mounted to replicate the form of an anterior

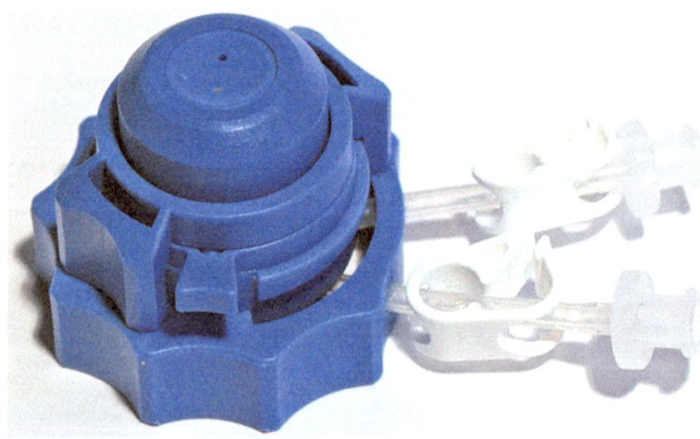

Fig. 3.16 Barron artificial anterior chamber (Katena)

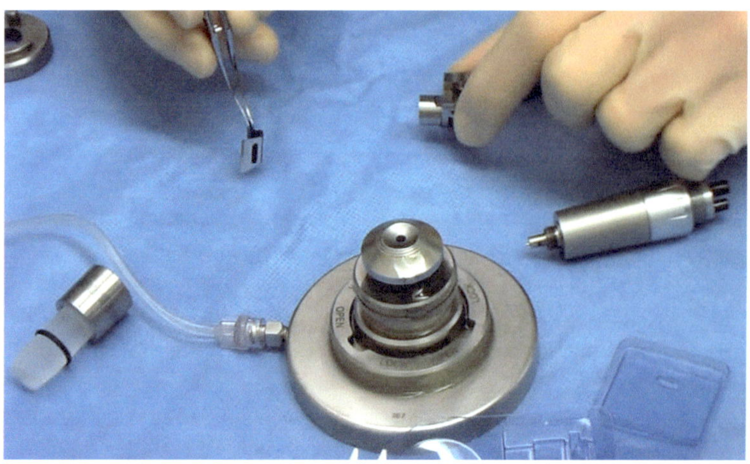

Fig. 3.15 Moria ALTK with blade, head, engine, artificial anterior chamber and tonometer (clockwise)

chamber. The corneo-scleral disc is secured onto the chamber by screwing down the plastic ring over the scleral rim. The chamber itself has two ports which can be connected to syringes containing air or fluid as required. The artificial AC is inflated with the desired fluid to a suitable pressure and the connecting tubing pinched closed. A lamellar dissection under the microscope can then proceed just as with a cornea in vivo. This is most often used in preparation of a posterior lamella for DSEK. Alternatively, it can be used with a suction trephine to cut a donor button for PKP or DALK from the epithelial side. Some surgeons favour this technique in a quest for better host-graft profile matching and reduced astigmatism.

3.4 Eye Banking

3.4.1 Tissue Retrieval and Preparation

Donor material is obtained from cadavers and must be harvested within 24 h of death. The management of donor material is often co-ordinated by local transplant coordinators after discussion with the deceased's family and consent has been obtained. In the UK, the Human Tissue Act 2004 and Act 2006 (Scotland) set out the requirements for specific consent for tissues to be retrieved, stored and used for transplantation and other specific purposes (training, education and research). Strict criteria must be met for tissue to be suitable for transplant before it is retrieved (Table 3.2).

Table 3.2 Suitability check list and criteria for corneal donor material

Infections	Previous surgery	Malignancy	Intrinsic eye disease	Others
HIV/AIDS	Immunosuppression	Leukaemia	Active ocular inflammation/uveitis	Death from unknown cause
Viral hepatitis (A, B or C)	Receipt of organ transplant	Lymphoma	Any congenital or acquired disorder of the eye	Suspect or confirmed
HTLV	Receipt of dura mater or brain surgery before 1992	Myeloma	Retinoblastoma	Creutzfeldt-Jakob disease
Seropositivity: anti-HIV, HBsAg, anti-HBc (if anti-HBs <100 IU/L), anti-HCV, anti-HTLV, syphilis	Receipt of human pituitary hormones	Polycythaemia	Malignant tumour of the anterior segment	Central nervous system diseases of unknown aetiology
Behaviour leading to risk of contracting HIV, hepatitis or HTLV1	Receipt of cornea, sclera or other human tissue allograft	Sideroblastic anaemia		Viral encephalitis or encephalitis of unknown origin, viral meningitis
Tattoos and body piercing within 6 months before death	Previous refractive laser surgery (LASIK and LASEK)	Myelodysplastic syndrome		Imprisonment within 12 months before death
Acupuncture within 6 months before death				
Bleeding disorders treated with blood-derived coagulation concentrates				
Rabies				
Congenital rubella				
Tuberculosis				
Reyes syndrome				
Progressive multifocal leukoencephalopathy				
Septicaemia				

After suitable training, tissue retrieval can be performed by ophthalmologists, specialist nurses and mortuary staff. The whole eye is removed and placed on an eye stand in a sterile pot containing a swab saturated with sterile saline. This forms a 'moist chamber' to protect the eye while in transit to the eye bank. The moist chamber is placed in an insulated box which also contains a sealed bag of melting ice to maintain a temperature of around 4 °C for 24 h. The sealed box is then sent by courier to one of the eye banks for processing.

A blood sample is required for virology screening; this must be ensured before the eye is retrieved. The donor material is screened for transmissible infections, particularly HIV, Hepatitis B and C, HTLV and syphilis. Unfortunately, there is no screening for Creutzfeldt-Jakob disease (CJD); hence, details of history act as exclusion criteria.

3.4.1.1 Modified Enucleation Protocol of the Royal College of Ophthalmologist (2008)

This protocol assumes use of an enucleation kit as provided in the Human Tissue Transport box, which is available free-of-charge through UK Transplant. Only single-use instruments are to be used.

1. Open eyelids and irrigate eyes with a sterile saline to remove debris, mucus and foreign matter. Clean face around the eyes, over eyelids, bridge of nose and eyebrows using alcohol wipes. Care should be taken not to touch the cornea with the alcohol wipes during this procedure.
2. Open the outer wrapper of a single-use instrument pack. Put on sterile gloves and place drapes and eye sheet over the donor.
3. Insert lid speculum and perform a peritomy using fine-toothed forceps and scissors. Tenon's capsule is pushed back by entering each of the four quadrants with the scissors and performing a blunt dissection.
4. Isolate the lateral rectus muscle with a muscle hook, insert artery forceps between hook and sclera and clamp muscle. Remove muscle hook and cut muscle distal but close to the clamp. Isolate and cut each of the remaining rectus muscles in turn, cutting with the scissors between the muscle hook and the sclera. There is no particular need to cut the oblique muscles. Care must be taken not to rub the cornea against the speculum or instruments.
5. Gently lift the eye with the artery forceps. Insert the enucleation scissors from the medial side, and, keeping the scissors almost vertical, locate the optic nerve by moving the scissors gently from side to side. Still keeping the scissors almost vertical, cut the optic nerve while maintaining gently upward pressure on the eye with the artery forceps. This should ensure that a stump of optic nerve at least 5 mm long remains attached to the eye.
6. Once the optic nerve has been severed, gently raise the eye from the orbit, excising residual tissue with the enucleation scissors.
7. Carefully transfer the eye to a plastic eye stand, passing the stump of the optic nerve through the hole in the base of the stand. Secure the eye on the stand by placing a sterile 25G hypodermic needle through the side of the optic nerve. Place the eye stand and eye (cornea uppermost) on top of a cotton wool ball (or gauze swab) moistened with saline in a sterile pot (moist chamber). The eye must not be immersed in any liquid in the moist chamber.
8. Remove the speculum and repeat the procedure with the other eye.
9. Pack orbits with cotton wool and, with the aid of eye caps, restore the original appearance of the donor.
10. Clearly label the moist chambers with the date, donor's name, date of birth, hospital and whether LEFT or RIGHT eye.
11. Pack the moist chambers and the blood sample into a Human Tissue Transport box. Fill a plastic bag with melting ice (at least 1 kg) and place bag into the box. Place completed Ocular Tissue Donor Information form and Retrieval Site Risk Assessment into the box. Contact the Duty Office at UK Transplant to report donor details and to arrange transport for the eyes.

3.4.2 Tissue Typing and Matching

Since the cornea is an immunologically privileged site, it differs from other tissues in the need to type donated material or match for HLA markers with the recipient. Studies in the 1990s did not show any survival benefit for HLA-matched corneas over non-matched grafts, but further work is underway for eyes receiving second grafts. There is some evidence that graft survival for high-risk or repeat grafts is higher with HLA-matched tissue. However, whenever possible, attempts are made to age-match donor and recipient within 30 years either way so that as far as possible a patient receives a cornea with a suitable endothelial cell density.

3.4.3 Tissue Preservation

At the eye bank the eye is assessed for suitability for transplantation. The intact globe is cleaned of adherent tissue and rinsed in sterile saline, then immersed in sterile polyvinylpyrrolidone 3 % solution (PVPI) for 3 min. After this it is placed in sodium thiosulphate 0.3 % to neutralise the PVPI before being rinsed in saline.

To excise the corneo-scleral disc, the eye is wrapped in a sterile gauze for ease of holding. A scleral incision is made with an 18 mm trephine taking care not to penetrate uveal tissue. This is extended around the circumference of the intended disc with scissors or scalpel, using the rounded end of the scissors to displace the ciliary body away from the cut. The disc can be gently teased away from the rest of the globe with forceps and placed anterior surface down in culture medium (e.g. GIBCO Minimum Essential Medium, Invitrogen Ltd, UK; or Optisol GS, DexSol and McCarey-Kaufman Media; Bausch & Lomb Surgical, Irvine, CA, USA).

The corneo-scleral disc is incubated in this culture medium containing an antibiotic and antimycotic cocktail for 1 week at 34 °C. A sample from the bottle is then taken to test for bacterial and fungal growth: 2 ml aliquots of the culture medium are transferred to a sterile universal tube and sent for microbiological assessment. Corneas that pass the microbiology, serology and history check can be released from quarantine. However, corneas can remain in this culture medium at 34 °C for up to 28 days (this is called organ culture condition). National Eye Banks in the UK only store under organ culture conditions. An alternative practice is 'cold storage' at 4 °C for up to 10–14 days. In the practice, fresh corneal tissue is not available (screening issues).

To assess suitability for transplantation, the endothelium is assessed for cell density and morphology. The corneo-scleral disc is placed epithelium-down in a petri dish, and a few drops of trypan blue are placed on the endothelium for 30 s and then washed off with sterile saline. Hypertonic sucrose (1.8 %) solution is added to the cornea to make the cell borders swell and make the cells easier to visualise. The cornea is viewed and photographed under sucrose at 100–120× magnification. The endothelial cell density (ECD) is recorded and the cell morphology assessed for regularity. The degree of folding is also assessed as cell death occurs along folds. In the UK, the minimal ECD is 2,200 cells/mm^2. Corneas with lower ECD are not used for penetrating keratoplasty but can be used for other types of surgery such as anterior lamellar keratoplasty. In the UK, only tissue unsuitable for transplantation can be used for training or research.

The cornea is then placed into a thinning medium (culture medium with 5 % w/v dextran T500, Fluka Analytical, Sigma-Aldrich Inc.) for a minimum of 6 h. Corneas are usually incubated for 24 h before sampling for microbial contamination again and then supplied for transplantation on day 3. Corneas may remain in medium containing dextran for up to 5 days and while in transport medium should not be refrigerated.

3.5 Penetrating Keratoplasty

Penetrating keratoplasty (PKP) is one of the most frequent and most successful organ transplantations (in the avascular cornea). A significant growth in frequency of PKP over the last decades can be attributed to better availability of graft material from establishment of eye banks and to better preservation media, allowing for maintenance of donor cornea for up to 4 weeks (culture). Further, the success of this operation has been improved by numerous advancements in the surgical technology and technique, including finer suture material, introduction of viscoelastic devices, new trephines and cutting blocks and improvements in antibiotic and anti-inflammatory drugs for the postoperative treatment (Figs. 3.17, 3.18, 3.19, 3.20, 3.21, 3.22, 3.23 and 3.24).

3.5.1 Technique

It is recommended that PKP is performed under general anaesthesia, especially for the beginner surgeon and more complex situations.

3.5.1.1 Preparation

Before the operation, the graft material is checked against the intended recipient and that the expiry date has not been exceeded. The transport media must be clear. The graft is placed endothelium-up on the cutting block and punched firmly with the trephine. Viscoelastic can be put onto the endothelium to prevent drying.

3.5.1.2 Corneal Marking

The centre of the host cornea is found and marked with a marker pen. A radial marker is centred on the cornea and used to place 8–10 ink marks on the recipient cornea to aid suture placement.

3.5.1.3 Trephination

Trephines are selected according to the desired graft size, taking into account the diameter and the disease of the recipient eye, for example, donor 7.75 mm and recipient 7.5 mm (see section 3.3.3.1). The (Barron) suction trephine is examined under the microscope to ensure the blade is smooth and free from scuffs or nicks which could prevent a clean incision. The blade is advanced to the point at which it will commence the cut, then withdrawn three quarter turns. The suction trephine is then applied to the recipient, taking care to centre it with respect to the markings and at equal distance from the limbus at all points, using the cross-hairs for assistance. It is better to take time over placement and then apply suction as this induces a groove in the cornea; if this is created in the wrong place, it is harder to locate the trephine securely in the correct place afterwards. Once the trephine is placed optimally, the blade is advanced to three quarter turns (count 1, 2, 3) to get into the cutting position. Continue rotating the blade and count again (1,2,3,...) for each quarter turn, which equals approximately 40–50 μm depth of cut per quarter turn. After eight turns, be even more careful and continue until there is full corneal penetration at one side (total of approx. ten turns). The suction is released immediately and the trephine is removed. Viscoelastic is placed into the open anterior chamber and remaining stromal attachments are incised with a blade or curved scissors.

3.5.1.4 Cardinal Sutures

Following clean removal of the host cornea, the prepared donor cornea is placed in position. For the first few sutures, the graft will be very mobile. The corneal button is hold with forceps (e.g. Pollack forceps) and 10/0 nylon is used to place four cardinal sutures which anchor the graft in place. The 12 o'clock suture is usually placed first, followed by the suture at 6 o'clock. Check

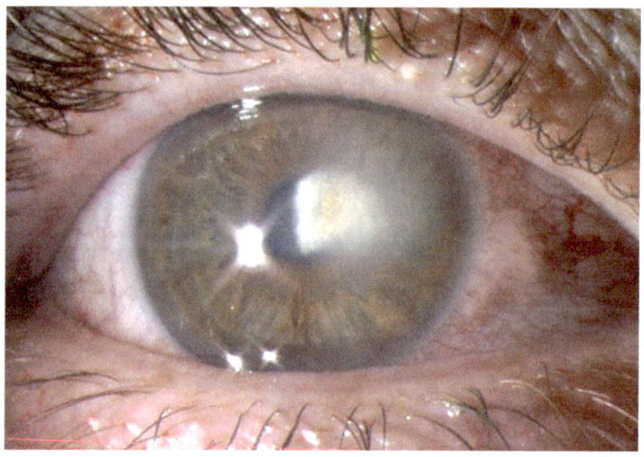

Fig. 3.17 Lipid keratopathy

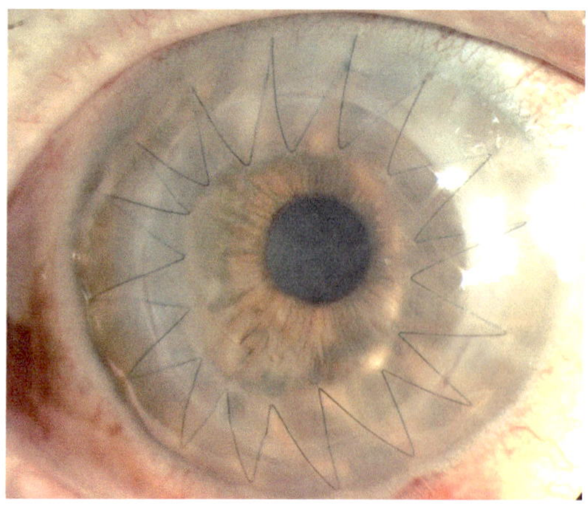

Fig. 3.18 One week after PKP with 16 bit continuous sutures (same patient as Fig. 3.17)

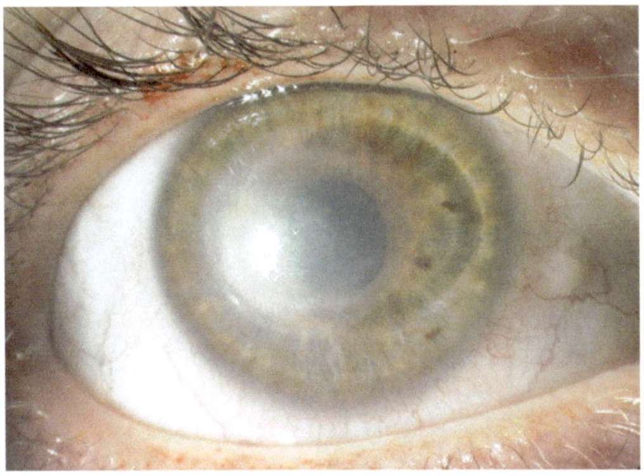

Fig. 3.19 Corneal scar after keratitis (acanthamoeba)

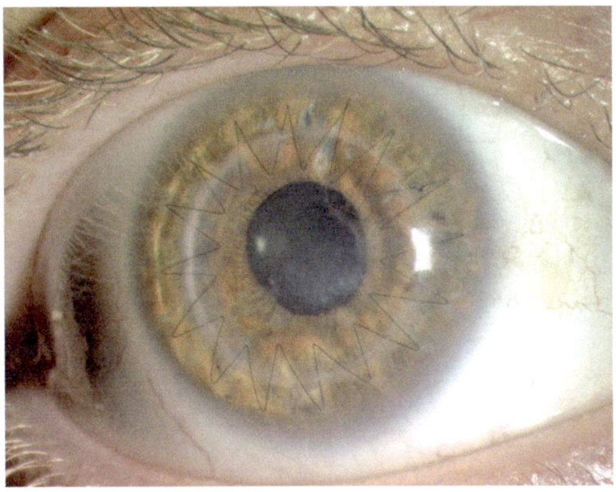

Fig. 3.20 Two months after PKP with 16 bit continuous sutures (same patient as Fig. 3.19)

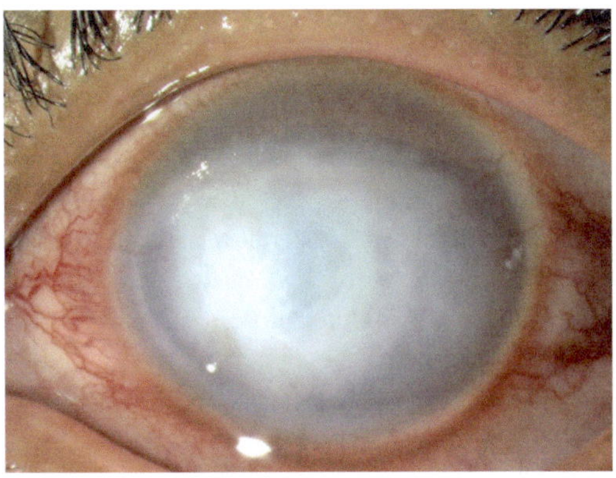

Fig. 3.21 Dense corneal scar after keratitis

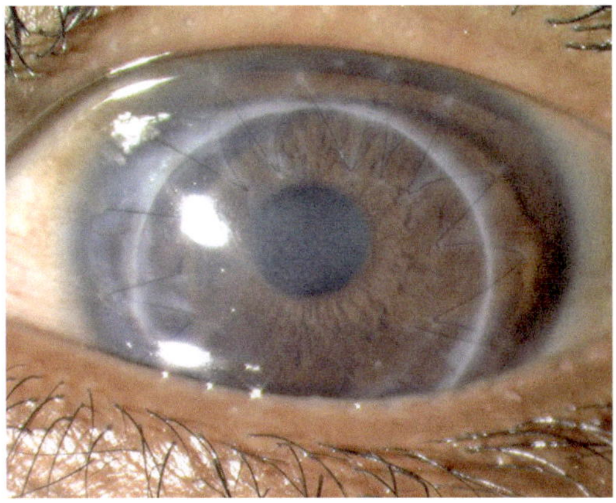

Fig. 3.22 Six weeks after PKP with 16 bit continuous sutures (same patient as Fig. 3.21)

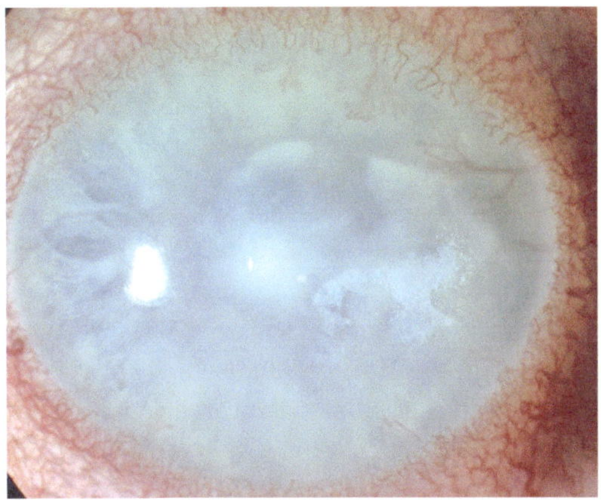

Fig. 3.23 Recurrent herpes simplex keratitis

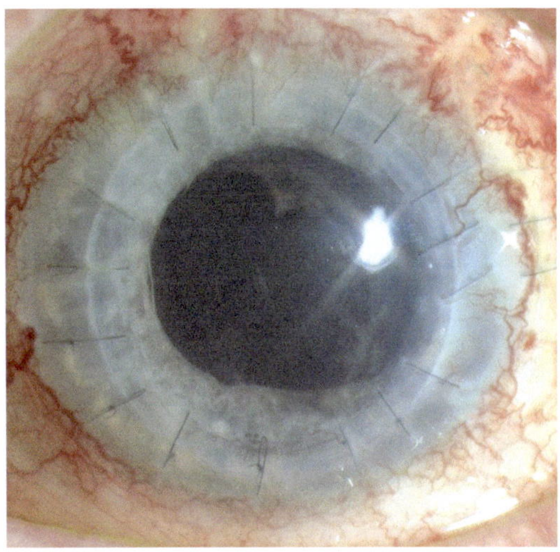

Fig. 3.24 Three weeks after PKP with interrupted sutures (same patient as Fig. 3.23)

Table 3.3 Important points suturing PKP

Cardinal sutures	Single interrupted suture (SIS)	Single continuous suture (SCS)
12 and 6, then 9 and 3	Indicated for paediatric keratoplasty, vascularisation in the host cornea, multiple previous rejections, inflammatory conditions and large grafts	Enabling postoperative suture adjustment as soon as cornea is re-epithelialised (ideally within 2–4 weeks)
Or: 11, 5 and 2, 8 position	Good for beginners, better apposition	Causing less inflammation if left more than 2 years
90 % depth, as close to the DM as possible	3-1-1, adjust the tension before second throw	At least 16 bites
The second suture is the most important	2-1-1, facilitate burial of the knot, tension adjustment more difficult	Commence tightening on the second or third bite to allow some laxity
Area of host/donor overlap should be equal	16 sutures is the average number	Bury knot at 12 o'clock
Nylon is more elastic and causes less stromal fibrosis	24–32 tighter sutures may be necessary in paediatric keratoplasty, same size graft and keratoconus	Cornea should be as spherical as possible
1mm bite on the graft and 1.5 mm on the host	Short ends, buried in host (less tension on the junction when ROS) or donor (reduced inflammation and vascularisation)	Remove scleral ring before adjustment of sutures Unpredictable suture-out astigmatism

graft alignment: the second suture is the most important and the areas of host/donor overlap should be equal. Check tension: sufficient tension is shown by formation of a bisecting groove in the cornea. Check depth: all sutures should be at 90 % corneal depth, as close to the DM as possible; the undercut recipient edge can be seen as a greyish line indicating where the needle should enter.

Inject Healon under the graft and continue with suturing at the 3 and 9 o'clock positions. The aim should be for as little manipulation as possible while placing secure sutures. After the first four sutures have been placed, the tension lines form a well-centred and regular diamond shape in the donor cornea.

Alternatively, adjustable or slip-knot sutures can be used to allow subsequent adjustment of tension; and some surgeons recommend to position the four sutures at 11, 5, 2 and 8 o'clock positions, as this may facilitate easier suturing. Six to eight cardinal sutures (=second cardinal suture) might be required in paediatric keratoplasty, if there is significant posterior pressure or in case of a thin donor or host.

All cardinal sutures can be removed after a continuous suture (Fig. 3.18) has been placed; but they might be left in place when the main sutures are interrupted.

Important points in relation to cardinal, single interrupted and single continuous suturing are summarised in Table 3.3.

3.5.1.5 Main Sutures

Further sutures are then placed according to the surgeon's preference (i.e. interrupted, continuous or a combination). If interrupted sutures are used, two or three more may be placed in each quadrant giving 12 or 16 in total (Fig. 3.24). The original cardinal sutures will probably appear loose at this stage and should be tightened. Finally, all suture ends must be rotated so that the knots are buried, preferably in the donor button, to reduce the risk of becoming vascularised and reduce the risk of rejection.

3.5.1.6 Finalising

Before tying the continuous suture tight, any viscoelastic remaining in the anterior chamber is removed with a Simcoe cannula and astigmatism can be assessed using a keratoscope or Morlet rule before securing the suture.

Once all sutures are tight, the AC should be reformed with balanced salt solution and the wound tested for leakage. The patient is given intradose of cefuroxime is 1mg in 0.1ml and sub-conjunctival betnesol 4 mg. Sub-Tenon's levobupivacaine 0.5 % (2–3 ml) can be given for pain relief if required. A bandage contact lens may be placed and the patient is reviewed the next day.

3.5.1.7 Aftercare

During the early postoperative period, the main goal is healing of the graft re-epithelialisation and avoidance of rejection and infection. Regular monitoring must include tonometry as glaucoma is both a complication of surgery (from structural changes induced by the surgery as well as induced by topical steroids) and a risk factor for graft failure. Later the attention should be directed towards visual rehabilitation.

Topical steroids are tapered slowly over the first 9–12 months. Refraction and corneal topography can guide selective suture removal if interrupted sutures were used.

Any remaining sutures should be removed around 12 months providing that sufficient healing has occurred at the graft-host interface to prevent dehiscence. Suture removal is usually done after topical steroids have been stopped, although a short course may be given after suture removal to prevent rejection.

3.5.2 PKP Triple Procedure

A patient with concurrent cataract undergoing penetrating keratoplasty may be suitable for simultaneous cataract extraction after excision of the diseased cornea ('open-sky technique'). The advantages of this include:

- Only requires one anaesthetic
- Reduces the risks of cataract surgery in the presence of corneal opacity
- Avoids the risk of graft rejection associated with cataract surgery after PKP

The disadvantages include:

- Greater risk of suprachoroidal haemorrhage due to increased length of time the eye is 'open'
- Less predictable refractive outcome
- More postoperative uveitis

If corneal clarity is sufficient, a continuous curvilinear capsulorhexis (CCC) may be created, with the use of vision blue, before trephination of the diseased cornea. It is preferable to create a CCC rather than a traditional 'can-opener' capsulotomy as the risk of radial capsule tear during nucleus removal is reduced and the subsequent IOL placement in the bag is more secure. If corneal opacity prevents CCC before removal of the corneal button, it may be achieved after this step in an 'open-sky' technique. Counterpressure on the anterior lens surface is required to oppose vitreous pressure and prevent tension forces from encouraging the capsulorhexis edge to tear out. This can be achieved by pressing on the anterior lens surface with a broad spatula.

Once the capsular opening is created, the lens nucleus can be removed. This was traditionally done by manual expression as in large incision ECCE surgery with pressure and counterpressure 180° apart at the limbus. However, a bulky lens may not pass easily through the CCC opening. One way to address this is to place a relieving incision in the capsular rim, but this may allow the CCC to tear out. A preferred alternative is to split the lens into two halves with a phaco chopper within the bag and remove the fragments through the intact opening.

Once the nucleus is completely removed, the cortex is cleared by an automated irrigation/aspiration (I/A) system or a manual aspiration method. With the automated I/A, little irrigation is required and the cortex can be engaged by gentle vacuum and peeled from the capsule. This is often difficult as the capsular bag is collapsed. The tip of the instrument can be used to hold the posterior capsule away from the aspiration port to prevent inadvertent aspiration and tear of the posterior capsule. If a manual aspiration cannula is used, it should have the aspiration port at the side of the tip rather than the end.

Finally, an intraocular lens can be inserted. A rigid (e.g. PMMA) or foldable three-piece lens (Acrysof MA60) may be preferable to a single-piece foldable lens as it will be more stable in the bag (or sulcus) and hold the posterior capsule and vitreous in place more effectively. The donor button can then be sutured in place in the usual way (see above).

3.5.3 Postoperative Refractive Error

When a stable refraction has been recorded, at least 4 weeks after removal of all sutures, spectacles or contact lenses may be prescribed.

Options for correction of higher refractive errors or irregular astigmatism include:

- Arcuate keratotomies, to reduce regular astigmatism. Various (less predictable) nomograms are available. Corrections of up to 4 D of astigmatism can sometimes be achieved.
- Compression sutures may be combined with orthogonal arcuate keratotomies for larger amounts of astigmatism.
- Excimer laser ablation (LASIK or LASEK) has become a treatment of choice for many surgeons to reduce small spherical refraction errors and astigmatism up to 4 D. LASEK is preferred to LASIK due to its greater predictability and the avoidance of flap-related complications. If LASIK is planned, a more accurate result may be obtained by a two-step procedure, that is, cutting the flap and allowing to heal before refracting and then planning the ablation profile as a separate procedure.
- Implantation of customised intraocular lens (phakic or pseudophakic) for correction of larger spherical refractive errors (>8 D) and regular astigmatism.

These procedures can be combined, for example, arcuate keratotomies to reduce large irregular astigmatism followed by excimer laser correction of the remaining ametropia.

3.6 Superficial Anterior Lamellar Keratoplasty

Superficial anterior lamellar keratoplasty (SALK) refers to selective replacement of anterior corneal stroma and epithelium with donor material. This is useful in cases such as superficial corneal scars, dystrophies limited to anterior stroma, or opacities resulting from previous refractive surgery. Tissue is removed to a depth comparable to a LASIK flap, that is, up to around 130 μm.

First, a donor corneal button is prepared using a microkeratome (or Femto-Laser) with a 130 μm blade to create a corneal lamellar graft of 9 mm diameter from a corneo-scleral transplant mounted on an artificial anterior chamber. Marking the anterior surface of the donor first helps prevent the graft being placed upside down as it may be difficult to orientate correctly.

The recipient cornea is prepared the same way, using a microkeratome to remove the anterior cornea (130 μm depth, 9 mm diameter). Any bleeding from cut vessels at the edge must be stopped with topical adrenaline as blood at the interface will compromise the visual outcome. The recipient bed should be cleaned.

The graft is then placed on the stromal bed where it adheres in a similar manner to a LASIK flap. The main difference is that there is no hinge so attachment is initially less secure. Overlay sutures keep the graft in place until it heals. 10/0 nylon sutures are passed over the periphery of the graft with bites only into host tissue, not into the graft itself. Conventional radial sutures should be avoided as they would apply uneven traction on the thin flap and cause significant astigmatism. Excess tension in the sutures should be avoided to prevent lifting of the graft edge. The interface can be irrigated and a bandage contact lens can be applied.

Visual recovery is usually rapid with little induced astigmatism. Sutures should be removed by 7 days as leaving them longer will create permanent 'stress lines' in the graft and may impede re-epithelialisation. The patient can be assessed for spectacles at 3 month post-op. Interface haze may limit visual acuity, but this tends to reduce over time.

The main benefits of this technique are removal of opaque tissue and the smoothing effect the procedure has on minor surface irregularities. Larger irregularities, however, may be reproduced in the stromal bed after the microkeratome cut. The procedure is risky if there are local corneal areas of thinning.

The host and graft tissue could alternatively be prepared with the femtosecond laser or by manual dissection.

3.7 Deep Anterior Lamellar Keratoplasty

Deep anterior lamellar keratoplasty (DALK) is the selective replacement of diseased stroma while retaining healthy Descemet's membrane (DM) and endothelium, for example, in patients with keratoconus. The aim is to remove all epithelium and stroma and expose DM as the bed for the graft; if a graft is placed onto host stroma, interface haze develops which limits vision.

Two main DALK techniques are established: 'Melles' technique' and 'big-bubble technique'. The relative merits of DALK versus PKP are shown in Table 3.4.

3.7.1 Melles' Technique

Melles described a technique for lamellar dissection close to Descemet's membrane for the removal of as much stroma as possible. General anaesthesia is preferred as patient movement can compromise achieving the lamellar dissection. The centre of the cornea and the intended graft size are marked, and a superior rectus stay suture is placed. A superior peritomy is made over 2 clock hours and careful cautery used to achieve haemostasis without distorting tissue. A deep scleral groove is made just posterior to the limbus, and a separate paracentesis is made to allow the anterior chamber to be filled completely with air.

Lamellar blades are introduced via the scleral groove, and the lamellar dissection is started. The air in the anterior chamber acts as a mirror and the reflection of the tip of the blade can be seen separated from the actual blade by twice the thickness of stroma remaining deep to the blade. The separation of images is used to guide the tip of the lamellar blade as close to Descemet's as possible without causing a perforation. Three blades are used which vary in length and profile, the longest having a pronounced convex curvature to allow the dissection to proceed over the apex of the cornea and to follow the corneal curvature beyond.

The dissection of keratoconic corneas in this way poses specific challenges:

- The corneal curvature may be exaggerated and be too steep for dissection to follow the desired plane.
- The apical cornea may be thin and fragile.
- Apical scarring from advanced keratoconus may lead to perforation in DM and prevent lamellar dissection.
- Previous hydrops may preclude clean separation of DM from stroma.
- Dissection of the cornea beyond the apex may be difficult because of the angle required to keep the blade tip close to the DM. Care must be taken here to avoid a shallow dissection plane.

Table 3.4 Comparison of deep anterior lamellar with penetrating keratoplasty

DALK	PKP
Technically more demanding	Shorter learning curve
Longer operation	Shorter anaesthetic required
Extra instruments required	Greater risk of endophthalmitis
Interface debris may remain and compromise vision	More likely to achieve vision of 6/6 at 12 months
Faster visual recovery	Suitable in presence of full-thickness pathology or deep scar
Earlier suture removal	
Fewer sutures	
Avoids risk of endothelial rejection	
Globe retains more structural integrity	
Reduced risk of intraoperative suprachoroidal haemorrhage	
Slightly less astigmatism	

Once the dissection has been achieved beyond the edges of the intended graft size, viscoelastic is introduced into the newly created plane, and some air is released from the anterior chamber to allow the remaining posterior lamella to be displaced posteriorly. The host tissue is trephined in the usual way.

Some stroma may remain if the dissection was not deep enough; this should be carefully excised as far as possible by lifting tissue carefully and cutting it free from DM with curved Vannas scissors. Thorough irrigation with BSS is used to remove any debris or viscoelastic. The bared DM must be as clean as possible as any debris captured in the interface may reduce visual potential.

To prepare the graft the donor cornea is placed endothelium-up on the trephine block as usual, but before punching the desired size donor, the DM and endothelium are removed. Trypan blue is used to stain the endothelium which is then removed centripetally by firm rubbing with a cellulose sponge or grasping with microforceps. Once all the DM/endothelium is removed, the graft is punched out as for a PKP and sutured onto the recipient.

Initially, four cardinal sutures are placed as for PKP and a continuous suture can be used to secure the graft. The suturing technique is slightly different in that the suture should pass at only 70 % depth in the graft and as deep into host stroma as possible (see diagram). The rationale for this is to compress the graft down onto the host DM to encourage healing.

Postoperatively, dexamethasone and antibiotic drops are given according to the surgeon's preference.

3.7.2 Big-Bubble Technique

Anwar and Teichmann described a technique for creating a cleavage plane between DM and stroma using air injected into the deep stroma (Figs. 3.25 and 3.26). High pressure is required to force air into the stroma and the air will find the path of least resistance. The attachment between DM and stroma is weaker than the inter-lamellar attachments within stroma so the injected air will preferentially separate tissue at this level.

The host cornea is first trephined to a preset partial-thickness depth (usually 60–80 % of corneal thickness). If available, this may be facilitated by using a femtosecond laser to create an incision which not only extends reliably to within 70 μm of DM but also has a sloping edge to facilitate access of instruments.

A 26G needle on an air-filled 3 ml syringe is introduced bevel-down into this groove and advanced 3–4 mm into mid-peripheral cornea. The needle tip must be placed in deep stroma without penetrating DM. Air is injected and as it is forced into the stroma it causes localised diffuse opacity. As injection continues, suddenly the air forms a large circular opacity with clear edges, indicating that a cleavage plane has been created between DM and stroma (the 'big bubble'). There is a loss of resistance at the plunger coincident with this which indicates the desired result. The edge should reach or exceed the trephined groove.

The stroma is removed in a lamellar fashion, leaving a thin layer over the bubble.

A paracentesis into the anterior chamber allows release of a small amount of aqueous. The bubble is then entered with the tip of a blade held parallel to the surface and a blunt-ended wire spatula advanced through this opening into the bubble. The surgeon then cuts down onto this to create a slit opening into the pre-DM space. This allows the remaining stroma to be lifted away from DM and excised with blunt-tipped microscissors. The exposed DM is irrigated to clear any debris ready for placement of the graft.

The preparation of the graft is the same as for the Melles' technique.

3.8 Posterior Lamellar Keratoplasty

In conditions causing endothelial dysfunction (e.g. Fuchs' endothelial dystrophy, aphakic or pseudophakic bullous keratopathy), selective replacement of Descemet's membrane (DM) and

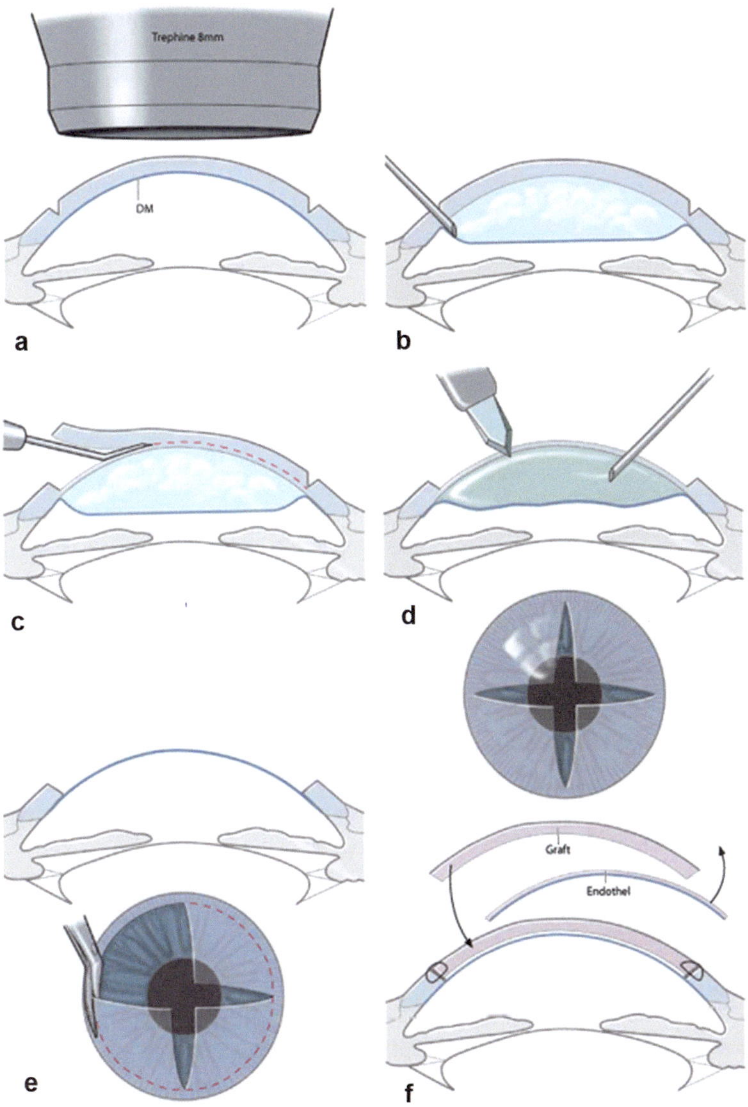

Fig. 3.25 Illustration of deep anterior lamellar keratoplasty (DALK) – big-bubble technique. (**a**) Partial thickness corneal trephine; (**b**) creating the big bubble by injecting air into the pre-Descemet's space; (**c**) lamellar dissection to remove superficial stroma; (**d**) entering the bubble with the blade and then filling the space with OVD; (**e**) excising the flaps of residual stroma leaving only DM and endothelium; (**f**) removal of DM/endothelium from the donor cornea and securing donor stroma with sutures

endothelium enables restoration of function with fewer of the risks associated with a penetrating keratoplasty.

The early approach to this was to create a donor lamella comprising endothelium, DM and a thin lamella of stroma (approx. 150 μm thick) and then remove a corresponding amount of tissue from the posterior corneal surface of the recipient to create a space into which to place the donor. This technique was termed deep lamellar endothelial keratoplasty (DLEK) but did not gain widespread acceptance because the posterior lamellar dissection of the host tissue was particularly difficult.

It was subsequently realised that removal of the host stroma was unnecessary and that once the host DM and endothelium had been removed the donor lamella would attach to the bared posterior surface of host stroma. This was termed Descemet's stripping endothelial keratoplasty (DSEK) and has become widely practised. When the donor lamella is prepared using a microkeratome rather than manual dissection, the term Descemet's stripping automated endothelial

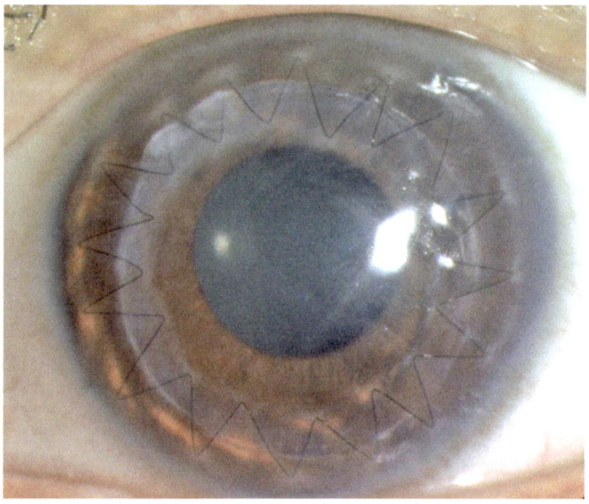

Fig. 3.26 One month after deep anterior lamellar keratoplasty (big-bubble technique)

Table 3.5 Comparison of Descemet's stripping endothelial keratoplasty techniques

DSEK	DSAEK
Microkeratome not required	Requires specific microkeratome (higher costs)
Longer learning curve to acquire skills for manual dissection	Smoother interface yields potentially better visual acuity
Longer operation	Grafts tend to be thicker
Theoretical greater risk of tissue wastage	
Less predictable graft profile	

keratoplasty (DSAEK) is used (Table 3.5), which increasingly makes DSEK obsolete.

3.8.1 Descemet's Stripping Automated Endothelial Keratoplasty

The donor cornea is prepared before the anaesthetic is given; in case the tissue cannot be prepared satisfactorily, the operation can be cancelled and postponed.

3.8.1.1 Donor Preparation (DSEK)

The donor cornea is mounted on an artificial anterior chamber (e.g. Barron) which is filled with air. Under the microscope a limbal incision

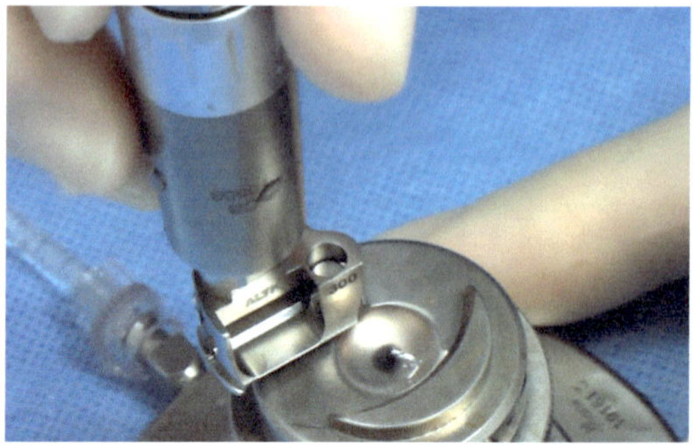

Fig. 3.27 Donor preparation with Moria ALTK cutting at 300 μm

is made with a guarded blade at 350 μm through 2 clock hours to guide the depth of the dissection. The surgeon performs a lamellar dissection aiming for a graft of approximately 150 μm. The same lamellar blades as used for DALK can be used, or if preferred a semi-sharp blade such as a Morlet lamellar dissector. Once the dissection is achieved, the graft is punched out from the endothelial side at the desired size (usually 8 mm) and then returned to the storage medium to minimise stress to the endothelial cells.

3.8.1.2 Donor Preparation (DSAEK)

The automated technique gives a more reliable thickness of posterior lamellar and better interface than manual dissection. The donor cornea is placed on the microkeratome's integrated artificial anterior chamber which is pressurised with balanced salt solution or viscoelastic (Fig. 3.27). One passage with the microkeratome blade removes the anterior portion of the cornea, leaving behind the posterior lamella. A corneal button is punched out with 8–8.5 mm diameter from the endothelial side and returned to the storage medium.

For the Moria microkeratome, the donor corneo-scleral disc must be between 16 and 19 mm in diameter. The epithelium is removed from the donor cornea and central pachymetry is performed. If the corneal thickness is less than 570 μm, a 300 μm microkeratome head is used; if the central corneal thickness is 570 μm or more, a 350 μm microkeratome head is used. Check the pressure of the mounted cornea before performing

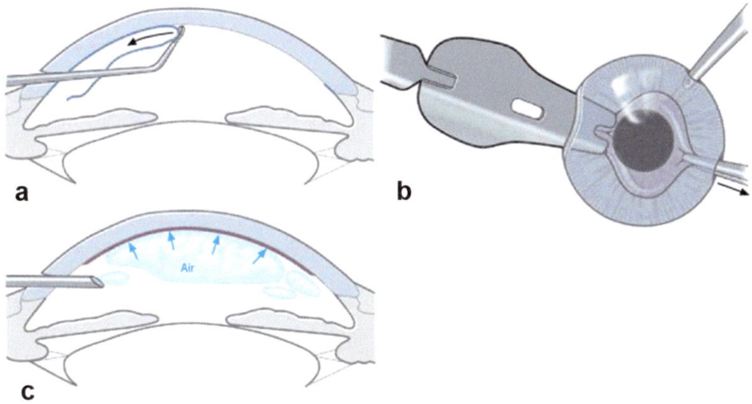

Fig. 3.28 Illustration of Descemet's stripping endothelial keratoplasty (and graft dehiscence). (**a**) Removing Descemet's membrane and endothelium; (**b**) introducing the donor lamella with the Busin glide and forceps; (**c**) tamponading the graft in place with air in the AC

the cut; it should be >65 mmHg (Barraquer tonometer: black ring within the white ring). Some surgeons mark the (anterior) corneal stroma after the cut and flap removal for orientation purposes.

3.8.1.3 Host Preparation

Surgery can be under peribulbar or sub-Tenon's block (often preferred to GA as patients are usually elderly). The pupil should not be dilated for surgery. A gentian violet ring mark is placed on the host epithelium to guide for same size removal of Descemet's membrane (ring marker size: 8–8.5 mm).

3.8.1.4 Main Incision and Paracentesis

A temporal limbal or (better) scleral tunnel is created with a width of 5 mm at 300 μm depth, 1–2 mm in length, and penetrated to the anterior chamber with a 3.2 mm keratome. Some surgeons construct smaller main incisions (3 mm instead of 5 mm) which have the advantage of self-sealing but the disadvantage of graft compression during insertion (endothelial trauma). Two paracenteses in a 90° angle both sides from the main incision are made, and the anterior chamber is filled with a cohesive viscoelastic.

3.8.1.5 Removal of Host Endothelium

A reversed Sinskey hook is used to separate the central from the peripheral endothelium the same size as marked with the ring marker (Fig. 3.28). The endothelium is then stripped from the stroma using the hook and Utrata forceps. The bared stroma around the periphery of this zone is scored gently with a bent 30G needle tip which increases the exposed surface area and enhances graft adherence. All viscoelastic is removed from the anterior chamber by irrigating with BSS and Simcoe, as any residual OVD at the interface will impair graft adherence.

3.8.1.6 Endothelial Graft Preparation

A small amount of OVD is placed on the endothelial side of the graft in preparation for insertion. Sometimes, orientation marks are placed on the stromal side of the graft. Fold the graft 2/3, bigger part on the top, and hold with insertion forceps, as used in cataract surgery.

3.8.1.7 Endothelial Graft Insertion

An anterior chamber maintainer is placed in one paracentesis and set at a low flow rate, and low bottle height maintains the anterior chamber without excessive fluid movement disturbing the unfolding of the graft. A peripheral iridectomy may be performed to prevent pupillary block glaucoma.

Several methods exist for insertion, all aiming to minimise the trauma to the endothelium to minimise cell loss (Table 3.6). The basic technique is similar to the implantation of a foldable intraocular lens using the insertion forceps (or Moria DSAEK forceps): the folded graft is held by the forceps and gently inserted through the main incision. Once the graft is inside the anterior chamber, the vacant paracentesis is used to inject air beneath the graft to unfold it in the correct orientation. The main incision is sutured with

Table 3.6 Techniques for endothelial graft insertion

Technique	Description
Forceps	The graft is folded endothelium-in to form a taco shape with a 2/3 overlap to aid orientation during unfolding (see text). Specially designed forceps with non-meeting tips are shaped so that the folded graft can be held with minimal pressure on the endothelium. The forceps also protect the graft against compression by the wound during introduction through the scleral tunnel
Pull-through	A 10/0 prolene suture (for IOL suturing) on a straight Ethilon needle (e.g. 15 mm, transchamber needle) is passed through the stroma of the graft (avoiding passing through the endothelium) at one edge and both ends of the suture (or one end following placing an overhand knot 4 cm away from the graft) are passed via the scleral tunnel across the anterior chamber and out through the cornea at the opposite limbus. Some surgeon place a small strip of OVD on the donor. The graft is then folded 2/3 (larger portion on the top) and pulled into the anterior chamber by the suture, taking care that it is not compressed as it passes through the scleral tunnel. Once the graft is positioned correctly, the suture is cut and withdrawn
Glides	Busin introduced a glide device comprising a gently curved section onto which the graft is placed and a tube through which the graft is delivered into the eye. The graft is placed endothelial side up on the loading section, then drawn into the tube with special microforceps. The tube is rotated so that when the graft is released inside the eye it will be oriented correctly. The glide is inserted into the main wound and the forceps are used via a paracentesis opposite to pull the graft from the glide into the anterior chamber. Again, the tube prevents compression of the graft as it travels through the wound. This device can be used with wounds as small as 3.2 mm
	Tan's endoglide is similar but folds the graft into a double-coil shape, with no touch between endothelial surfaces. The graft is loaded into the glide which is inverted and inserted through the wound. The graft is held in position with special microforceps in position as the glide is withdrawn. Tan has also described the use of a modified Sheet's glide (as used in cataract surgery). The donor lenticule is placed endothelial side down on viscoelastic on the glide which is inserted into the anterior chamber. The graft is then drawn into position with forceps inserted as above through a paracentesis opposite the main wound. This has the advantages of not folding/unfolding the graft, which reduces endothelial trauma, and no chance of the graft unfolding upside down. A larger wound (5 mm) is needed
Injectors	These devices are similar to injectors for intraocular lenses. The Endosaver (Ocular Systems Inc) has a carrier onto which the graft is placed endothelium-up and which folds the graft as it is retracted into the barrel. The barrel is rotated and inserted into the AC, and as the barrel retracts the graft is released. This is suitable for grafts up to 8.5 mm diameter and 175 μm thick and requires a wound of at least 4 mm

10/0 nylon; the anterior chamber maintainer can be removed.

3.8.1.8 Graft Placement and Fixation

The endothelial graft is centred by stroking the corneal surface with a Rycroft cannula ('corneal massage'). This also encourages egress of fluid from the graft-host interface. Further air is added to the anterior chamber to raise the pressure (40 mmHg) with the aim of compressing the graft against host stroma and encouraging adhesion. Some surgeons favour pre-placing paracentral penetrating slit incisions earlier in the procedure so that at this stage any fluid at the graft-host interface will be displaced out through the slits to reduce the risk of later graft dehiscence. A custom roller device may be used on the corneal surface to massage out any interface fluid. This high pressure is maintained for 10 min, after which time most air is released carefully to allow the IOP to normalise while retaining a sufficient (small) bubble to keep the graft in position.

3.8.1.9 Finalising

The paracenteses are sutured with 10/0 nylon. Sub-conjunctival betamethasone 2 mg and cefuroxime 125 mg are given. The speculum must be removed very carefully to avoid distorting the cornea as this may increase the risk of failure of graft adherence. The patient remains in a face-up position for atleast 2 h as they leave the operating theatre to return to the ward. The IOP should be

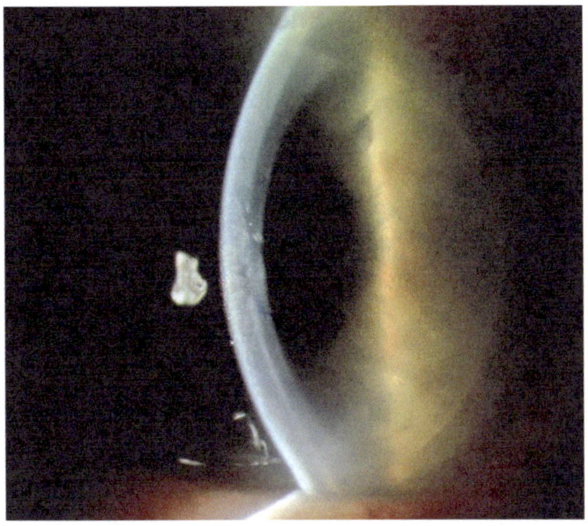

Fig. 3.29 One week after Descemet's stripping keratoplasty

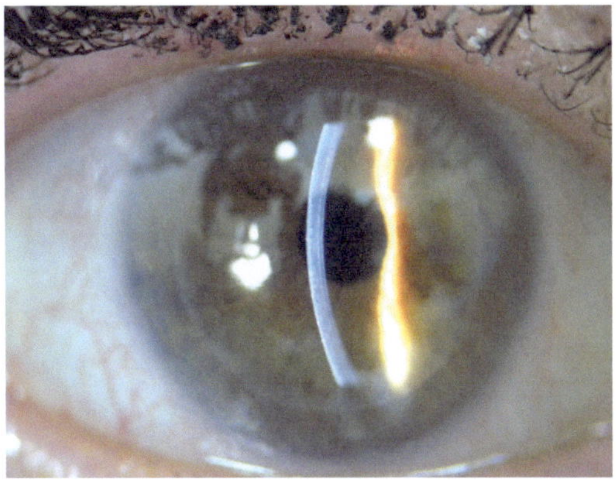

Fig. 3.31 One year after Descemet's stripping keratoplasty (overview)

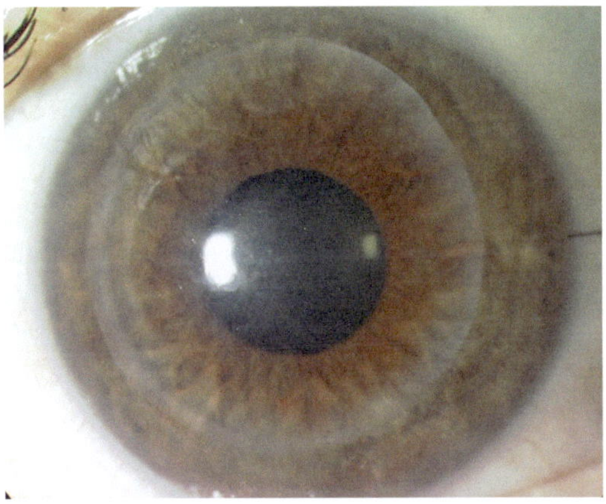

Fig. 3.30 Three months after Descemet's stripping keratoplasty

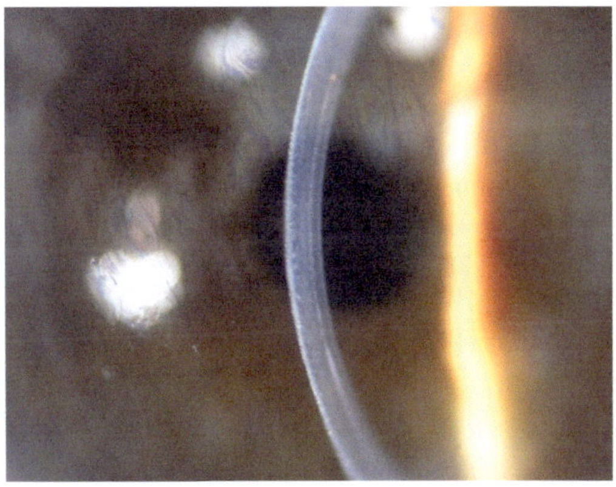

Fig. 3.32 One year after Descemet's stripping keratoplasty (slit; same patient as Fig. 3.30)

measured before the patient is discharged and the graft checked for adherence.

3.8.1.10 Postoperative Management

Postoperatively the patient is given a reducing regime of topical steroid according to the surgeon's preference (Figs. 3.28, 3.29, 3.30, 3.31 and 3.32). Some surgeons aim to stop the topical steroid completely after this; others prefer for the patient to take a very low daily maintenance dose of a weak steroid indefinitely (e.g. fluorometholone once daily). This is unlikely to induce glaucoma and reduces the risk of rejection without the compromise in tissue healing which this would risk in PKP or DALK.

3.8.2 Descemet's Membrane Endothelial Keratoplasty

Descemet's membrane endothelial keratoplasty (DMEK) represents the natural evolution of selective posterior lamellar keratoplasty. Transplantation of just the endothelium and Descemet's membrane (DM) brings the benefits of selective endothelial transplantation but avoids the complications associated with implanting stroma. The technique is still evolving and is offered by a limited number of specialist centres. Advantages and disadvantages of DMEK are shown in Table 3.7.

Table 3.7 Advantages and disadvantages of Descemet's membrane endothelial keratoplasty

Advantages of DMEK	Disadvantages of DMEK
Less haze from stroma-stroma interface	Technically harder
Better visual potential	More likely to damage tissue by manipulation
Reduced refractive shift	More likely to lose ECD
Experiential outcome data	Less clinically proven
Faster visual rehabilitation	Risk of tissue wastage during dissection
Larger area of DM/endothelium transplanted (including peripheral cornea where ECD is greater) so overall higher number of endothelial cells	

3.8.2.1 Preparing the Host

The recipient eye is prepared in the same way as for DSEK with removal of a disc of diseased endothelium to bare the recipient stromal bed. A smaller incision (3.5 mm) can be used as less tissue is to be implanted.

3.8.2.2 Preparing the Graft

The graft is prepared by securing the donor corneo-scleral disc endothelium-up on a specially designed suction mount. Using a hockey stick blade the, edge of DM is loosened just anterior to the trabecular meshwork and scleral spur around 180° of the circumference. The DM is gently pushed centrally, loosening its attachment. The edge can then be picked up with microforceps and the DM/endothelium sheet stripped from stroma until about ½ to 2/3 is free. This sheet is replaced back onto its original position by immersion in saline in preparation for trephination. A 9.5 mm trephine is applied to cut just into posterior stroma. The previously freed edge of this 9.5 mm disc is grasped again with the forceps, and the DM is completely stripped from the stroma. Due to the elastic properties of the tissue, the stripped endothelium/DM rolls spontaneously with the endothelium always on the outside. This helps with orientation of tissue during implantation.

3.8.2.3 Implantation Process

To aid visualisation the endothelium roll is stained with trypan blue and sucked up into an injector device (e.g. a custom-made device (Hippocratech, Rotterdam) or one designed for implantation of the implantable collamer lens (Staar Surgical, Monrovia, Ca)). The device can be filled with balanced salt solution (BSS) or a hydroxypropyl-methylcellulose preparation (Ocucoat, B&L) to support the graft. This is then introduced through the wound and the endothelium is injected.

3.8.2.4 Placing the Graft at the Host Site

Unrolling the graft may be difficult. This can be achieved by ensuring the graft centrally with the rolls upwards and injecting bursts of BSS to begin unrolling it. Maintaining a shallow anterior chamber helps at this stage to prevent the scroll from reforming. A small air bubble is then injected to keep the graft in place and encourage the graft to unroll completely. Alternatively, the graft can be spread out on the iris and a bubble of air injected under the graft to lift it up into place against the bared stroma. The duration of the air fill at the end of surgery may need to be longer than for DSEK/DSAEK. Typically the anterior chamber is completely filled for 30–40 min before controlled partial air/fluid exchange.

3.8.2.5 Complications

Complications of DMEK are summarised in Table 3.8.

3.8.2.6 DMAEK

This is a combination of microkeratome-prepared posterior lamella, and further dissection with a big-bubble technique allows preparation of a Descemet's membrane/endothelial graft with a thin rim of stroma around its edge. This combines the advantages of the DM/endothelium graft with easier handling and more predictable unfolding once in the anterior chamber.

3.8.3 DSAEK Triple Procedure

Posterior lamellar surgery (DSEK, DSAEK) can be combined with phacoemulsification as a new triple procedure. The advantages of this include

Table 3.8 Complications of Descemet's membrane endothelial keratoplasty

Complications of DMEK
Tearing of Descemet's membrane during graft preparation. If the tear is outside the central 9 mm zone, the tissue may be salvageable and used to prepare a DSAEK or DSEK graft instead
Partial or complete graft dislocation. Usually seen within the first few days (up to 2 weeks) after surgery. Can be managed by rebubbling
Primary graft failure
Glaucoma (up to 15 % of cases) from pupil block caused by the air bubble or secondary to topical steroids. Pupil block can be prevented by preoperative YAG-laser peripheral iridotomy or relieved by pupil dilatation and/or releasing air via a paracentesis if it is encountered
Rejection is unusual but may be seen in around 3–10 % of cases (more common in Asian recipients than Caucasians) and is usually reversible with intensive topical steroids

needing only one procedure and rapid visual rehabilitation. Disadvantages include difficulty with refractive prediction and greater likelihood of refractive surprise, more postoperative inflammation and greater risk of graft failure. The combination also lengthens the procedure so a long-acting local anaesthetic agent such as levobupivacaine must be considered for the initial block.

3.9 Aftercare

3.9.1 Treatment and Follow-Up

Patients require careful and frequent follow-up after surgery since complications, if not detected and managed appropriately, can cause graft failure and reduce the chance of success in future keratoplasty. Patients must be aware of this aspect of their care before they embark on surgery. If they are not able or willing to attend for follow-up, keratoplasty should be avoided. Patients also have to understand that symptoms suggestive of infection or rejection (pain, photophobia, redness, reduced vision) should be treated as a sight-threatening emergency, sometimes requiring hospital admission. Patients should be given emergency contact telephone numbers so that they can request an urgent review should they have any problems.

Table 3.9 Topical treatment after keratoplasty

Standard treatment (low risk, e.g. first corneal graft for keratoconus)	Intensive treatment (high risk, e.g. host eye with ocular surface inflammation)
G. chloramphenicol 0.5 % preservative free qds for first 3 weeks	G. chloramphenicol 0.5 % preservative free qds for first 3 weeks
G. dexamethasone 0.1 % preservative free qds for first 4 weeks; then preserved qds for 4 weeks, tds for 4 weeks, bd for 4 weeks, daily for 4 weeks; then G. fluorometholone 0.1 % qds for 4 weeks, tds for 4 weeks, bd for 4 weeks and daily for 4 weeks; then stop	G. dexamethasone 0.1 % preservative free qds for first 4 weeks; then G. prednisolone sodium phosphate 0.5 % tapering as qds for 4 weeks, tds for 4 weeks and bd for 4 weeks; then daily as long as required

3.9.1.1 Priorities During Follow-Up After Keratoplasty

1. Prevention, detection and treatment of infections
2. Management of new or pre-existing co-pathologies, especially glaucoma
3. Visual rehabilitation with treatment of existing refractive errors

3.9.1.2 Topical Treatment (Steroids and Antibiotics)

Patients are prescribed topical steroid and antibiotic eye drops after surgery. A bandage contact lens may be used. The exact regime will depend on the surgeon's practice and the risk stratification of the case, whether it is a primary graft or a repeat procedure and whether there was any preoperative corneal neovascularisation (Table 3.9).

3.9.1.3 Removal of All Sutures (ROS)

For penetrating keratoplasty, suture removal is typically around 12 months after surgery, whereas after DALK sutures can be removed earlier, around 9 months post-op. Some surgeons prefer to leave sutures in for longer (up to 18 or 24 months), especially in elderly patients, unless removal is necessary for visual rehabilitation.

Some surgeons aim to stop topical steroid before suture removal, others continue low-dose steroid until after sutures are removed. Assessment of the degree of healing should precede suture removal since there is a risk of dehiscence if the graft-host interface is weak. This is more likely to be the case in older patients or those taking long-term topical or oral steroids. In such patients it may be safer to leave sutures indefinitely and maintain vigilance for suture-related problems such as breakage or infection. A strong fibrous ring at the graft-host interface indicates sufficient healing has occurred.

Sutures can be removed at the slit lamp, but if a removal of an interrupted suture or large number of interrupted sutures is planned, it is often more comfortable for patient and surgeon if this is done under the operating microscope. Once all sutures are removed, the patient should be reviewed within a couple of days to check for leakage or wound gap, and at 6 weeks with refraction and corneal topography to plan correction of refractive errors with contact lenses or spectacles.

3.9.1.4 Selective Removal of Corneal Sutures

Selective suture removal can be considered as part of the visual rehabilitation process to reduce astigmatism. This should be guided by subjective refraction and topography. Patients should receive topical antibiotic and steroid cover for 1–2 weeks after suture removal to reduce the risk or precipitating infections or rejection.

3.9.1.5 Broken or Loose Sutures

Broken or loose suture must be removed as soon as they are identified as they trap mucus in the tear film, become vascularised and become a focus for infection or rejection.

3.9.1.6 Re-suturing

After removal of sutures if the graft-host interface has not healed sufficiently, there is a risk of slippage or even dehiscence. If this is observed the graft will need to be re-sutured.

3.9.2 Additional Treatment and Medication

3.9.2.1 Management of Glaucoma

Glaucoma is a specific complication of corneal graft surgery and is probably multifactorial in cause. Estimates for the incidence of post-keratoplasty glaucoma range from 9 to 35 %. Potential causes of post-keratoplasty glaucoma include:

- Intraocular inflammation – fibrinous uveitis, peripheral anterior synechiae, posterior synechiae
- Structural changes in the iridocorneal angle by long or deep suture bites
- Collapse of trabecular meshwork
- Retained viscoelastic
- Topical steroids
- Pupil block (in DSEK/DSAEK)
- Aqueous misdirection

Glaucoma is a specific risk factor for graft failure so it is doubly important to monitor for this and treat aggressively. This is made more difficult especially in the early post-keratoplasty phase due to:

- Difficulty measuring IOP: Irregular corneal surface makes Goldman tonometer mires difficult to identify and interpret; central corneal thickness may initially be increased by oedema; large amounts of astigmatism may make it difficult to know how best to orient the mires (horizontally or obliquely); poor toleration of contact tonometry by patient with inflamed eye
- Poor view of the optic nerve
- Unreliable fields due to difficulty of correcting for near vision or poor corrected vision
- Physician distraction: Preoccupation with the state of the cornea, stage of healing and visual rehabilitation
- Patients' compliance: Confusion with the management of many different eye drops at different times

Glaucoma assessment and monitoring post-keratoplasty can be improved by making IOP measurements part of the protocol:

- If Goldman tonometry mires are distorted, a Tonopen is a reliable and well-tolerated alternative.
- If the patient cannot perform perimetry but the view of the disc is reasonable, sequential OCT scans of the optic disc and retinal nerve fibre layer are a reliable way of detecting structural changes in the optic nerve head and may flag up development or progression of glaucoma.
- Most patients will benefit from having written instructions about which drops to take and when.

Glaucoma should be treated initially with topical medication, ideally in a preservative-free form. In the UK, a prostaglandin analogue, beta-blocker and carbonic anhydrase inhibitor (CAI) are available as preservative-free preparations. If this is insufficient, filtration surgery may be required, for example, trabeculectomy or tube/valve implantation. Lamellar corneal surgery often requires a scleral tunnel approach which may result in conjunctival scarring, which in turn can increase the risk of failure of subsequent glaucoma surgery. Such cases should therefore be considered high risk and may be better managed in collaboration with a glaucoma specialist.

Pupil block after DSEK is caused by the air bubble in the anterior chamber. It can be prevented by avoiding leaving the eye overfilled with air at the end of the procedure, and by performing an inferior peripheral iridectomy at the time of surgery (or a YAG-laser iridotomy before surgery). If it does develop it can be treated by dilating the pupil and releasing a small volume of air from the AC via the paracentesis if necessary.

3.9.2.2 Management of Herpetic Eye Disease

Patients with a history of herpes simplex keratitis (HSK) undergoing corneal grafting pose a number of additional problems. There may be pre-existing reduction in corneal sensation, dry eye and corneal neovascularisation, all of which reduce the chance of graft survival.

The corneal environment must be optimised preoperatively with lid hygiene measures and topical lubricants. Prominent corneal vessels may be amenable to fine needle diathermy or argon laser photocoagulation. Deep stromal vessels increase the risk of subsequent graft rejection. Keratoplasty should ideally only be performed after the keratitis has been quiescent for at least 6 months. Prophylactic oral acyclovir should be considered.

Postoperatively the patient should receive prophylactic oral acyclovir 400 mg bd as well as the usual regime of topical antibiotic and steroid. The acyclovir and topical steroid may need to be continued for around 12 months. Alternatives to acyclovir are valacyclovir 500 mg once or twice daily or famciclovir 125–250 mg twice daily.

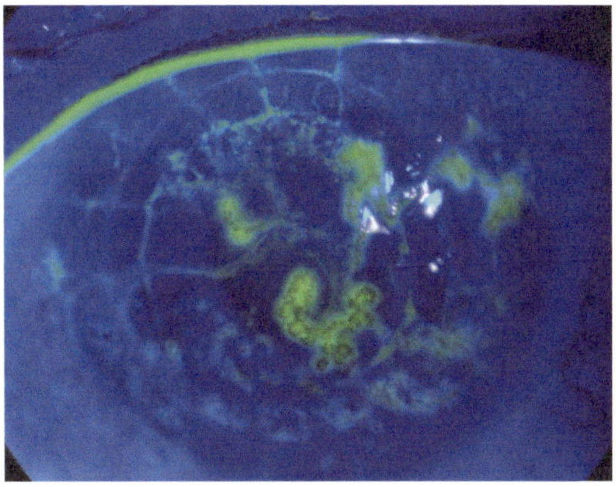

Fig. 3.33 HSV reactivation (fluorescein stain) on the corneal graft

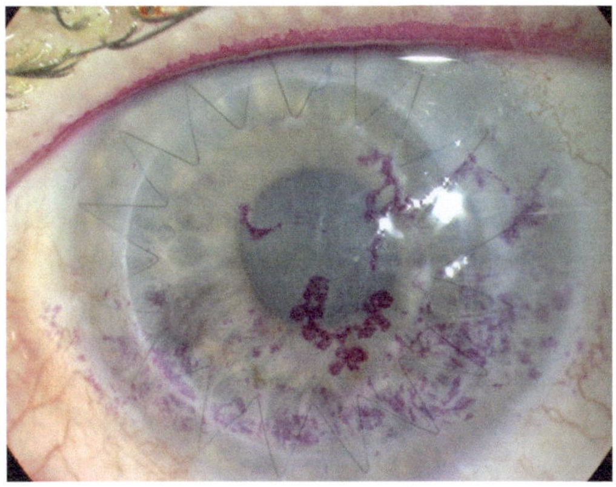

Fig. 3.34 HSV reactivation (Bengal Rose stain) on the corneal graft (same patient as Fig. 3.33)

Reported incidences of recurrence of HSK after penetrating keratoplasty range from 15 to 47 %.

Reactivation of virus (Figs. 3.33 and 3.34) may occur in the graft, but graft failure may also be caused by herpes simplex virus in the absence of prior known disease. This is likely to be due to latent viral infection of either host or donor cornea. Reactivation may be difficult to differentiate from rejection, but the clinician should look out for dendritic ulcers or large keratitic precipitates with donor and recipient corneal oedema. Treatment with topical steroid and antiviral should be initiated. Recurrence of HSK in the graft increases the chance of graft rejection or failure. Rejection rates of 29 % in 1 year and 46 % in 2 years were reported, but graft survival was still reasonable (84 % at 1 year and 67 % at 2 years). The need for regrafts in eyes with HSK has reduced over the last few decades due to the improvement in medical treatment of HSK (50 % in the 1970s, 22 % in the 1980s and 6 % in the 1990s) and patient selection.

3.10 Complications

3.10.1 Intraoperative Complications of PKP

3.10.1.1 Eccentric Trephination

Eccentric trephination is a risk if insufficient care is taken when positioning the trephine or if the corneal curvature is highly irregular, for example, in severe keratoconus. The centre of the cornea should be marked carefully before the trephine is placed and the cross hairs of the trephine placed over the mark. The distance from the trephine to the limbus in several meridia can also be used as an aid to centration. The best position for the trephine must be chosen before vacuum is applied since this creates a furrow in the cornea, and if the surgeon wishes to reposition the trephine after this stage, it may be difficult to prevent the trephine from returning to this original position. Insufficient vacuum during trephination can allow the trephine to slip and create an asymmetric recipient site. Eccentric trephination is likely to induce astigmatism or other visual aberrations such as coma; it also shows an increased risk for rejection.

3.10.1.2 Retained Descemet's Membrane

In oedematous corneas, for example, pseudophakic bullous keratopathy, the lamellae of the host may be easily separated and the trephine may separate Descemet's membrane from stroma, displacing it posteriorly rather than cutting it and creating a pseudo-anterior chamber. If scissors are used to complete the host excision, the retained Descemet's membrane may be pushed further away from the stromal rim. If this is not recognised, when a full-thickness donor button is sutured in place, there will be severe damage to the donor endothelium resulting in graft failure. Retained DM must be checked for before placement of the donor and excised if necessary with a diamond blade or scissors.

3.10.1.3 Suprachoroidal Haemorrhage (± Expulsion of Ocular Contents)

This devastating complication is fortunately rare (<0.5 %). Risk factors include atherosclerosis, increased age, hypertension, glaucoma, anticoagulant therapy and local anaesthetic surgery. Patients with reduced compliance, for example, not understanding the language, difficulties in keeping still or severe cough, are also at higher risk. Risk factors should be assessed and addressed as much as possible. The initial penetrating incision into the eye should be made cautiously to avoid a precipitous drop in intraocular pressure and the eye left open for as little time as possible. If an expulsive haemorrhage is suspected (appearance of a dark choroidal detachment or anterior movement of ocular contents), closure of the eye must be achieved as quickly as possible, perhaps with a finger if necessary. Posterior sclerostomy to allow drainage of the haemorrhage may be considered if repositioning of ocular contents and formation of an anterior chamber cannot be achieved. Once this could be stabilised, the eye should be closed completely and any protruded material should be placed back into the eye. Generally, the visual outcome is very bad and the chance for developing secondary glaucoma is high.

3.10.1.4 Inappropriate Trephine Choice

If trephines are chosen poorly or mixed up, a graft too small for the recipient opening may be cut. If the recipient has not yet been trephined, a more suitable trephine size can be substituted. If the recipient has already been trephined, the graft should be sutured in place taking extra care to ensure no wound leak at the end of the procedure. A greater degree of ametropia may be expected, particularly hypermetropia. The tight sutures required to close the wound are also more likely to distort the iridocorneal angle and induce postoperative glaucoma. It may be necessary to replace the graft with a more appropriately sized graft subsequently. In extreme cases, the trephined host cornea may be used to close the eye temporarily instead of the undersized donor cornea.

3.10.1.5 Damage to Crystalline Lens (Phakic Patient)

Inadvertent contact between instruments and the anterior lens capsule can induce cataract in a phakic patient, especially if the capsule is penetrated. The pupil should be constricted preoperatively with pilocarpine 2 % eye drops to protect the lens. Controlled entry into the eye and careful instrument handling reduce the risk of accidental contact and damage.

3.10.1.6 In Relation to the Sutures (Location)

Bites that are too long increase the risk of glaucoma, vascularisation and rejection, especially if too close to the limbus. Very short bites are difficult to rotate and may not hold the tissue securely in place. Sutures that are too tight or loose can induce astigmatism and are at risk of dehiscence. Bites that are not placed radially (perpendicular to the cut) induce torque and astigmatism. Very shallow bites allow posterior wound gape, and bites that are too deep may penetrate the cornea and increase the risk of endophthalmitis.

3.10.1.7 In Relation to a Continuous Suture

A continuous suture can break before completion; the ends then can be tied together, but this will create two knots in the final suture, and it may be difficult to ensure that both knots are buried without uneven tension. Special care must be exercised in manoeuvring the needle as contact between the tip and forceps will blunt the needle and make subsequent sutures passes difficult. If excessive turning force is applied through the needle during passes, it can be easily bent. Use of a double-ended suture allows the suture to be completed in the other direction if one needle should become unusable.

3.10.2 Intraoperative Complications of DALK

3.10.2.1 Perforation of the Descemet's Membrane During Dissection

Dissection too deep with Melles' technique risks causing a perforation in the Descemet's membrane. If this is very small and peripheral, it may be possible to continue with the DALK, but a larger perforation may require converting to penetrating keratoplasty. If there is an inherent weakness in the Descemet's membrane, the pressure generated during big-bubble creation may tear the Descemet's membrane at the weak point and necessitate conversion to a penetrating procedure.

3.10.2.2 Full-Thickness Trephination

If the Descemet's membrane is not adequately displaced posteriorly, the trephine may advance beyond stroma and perforate the membrane. This can be managed by either converting to penetrating keratoplasty or closing the keratotomy incision and allowing at least a month for the Descemet's membrane to heal. After the waiting time, DALK can be attempted again by lamellar dissection.

3.10.2.3 Dissection Too Shallow

Failure to remove adequate stroma will lead to interface haze when the graft heals. This does fade in time but risks reducing the visual potential.

3.10.2.4 Inadequate baring of the Descemet's Membrane

Failure to clear the Descemet's membrane of stroma after big-bubble creation and stromal excision may also result in interface haze. There is a fine balance between clearing as much stroma as possible and risking a perforation.

3.10.2.5 Failure to Achieve Big Bubble

Air may leak into the stroma, back along the needle entry track or through trabecular meshwork into the anterior chamber. As air enters the stroma, it becomes opaque and limits the view for further attempts to create a big-bubble and lamellar dissection. Two or three attempts at creating a big bubble may be possible (at different positions around the cornea), but if these fail it is necessary to remove stroma by serial lamellar dissections.

3.10.2.6 Air Entry into the Anterior Chamber via Trabecular Meshwork

During big-bubble formation, instead of separating the stroma from the Descemet's membrane, the air may track through the stroma via trabecular meshwork into the anterior chamber. The surgeon may try to create a big bubble from another starting point around the incision. It is unclear whether this damages the trabecular meshwork and makes postoperative glaucoma more likely.

3.10.2.7 Interface Debris or Blood

Any debris remaining at the graft-host interface may reduce the final visual potential. Thorough irrigation of the host bed should therefore precede placement of the donor button. Persistent bleeding from vessels in the recipient stroma should be addressed with micro-cautery (taking care not to distort the stromal rim) or topical phenylephrine or adrenaline.

3.10.2.8 Sutures Too Shallow or Penetrating

Poor placement of sutures can increase the amount of postoperative astigmatism. Since recipient Descemet's membrane remains in situ there is less of a need to create watertight wound closure and sutures do not need to be as tight as for PKP. However, optimal suture tension and placement should be pursued as this will give a better postoperative refractive outcome.

3.10.3 Intraoperative Complications of DSEK

3.10.3.1 Donor Tissue Damaged While Dissecting

Preparation of the posterior lamellar disc requires a certain degree of manipulation during which endothelial damage may be sustained. Manual dissection at too deep a level may perforate the Descemet's membrane. Manipulation of tissue to position the disc on the artificial anterior chamber may damage endothelial cells. While the tissue is out of storage medium, the endothelial cells are exposed to metabolic stress; this time should be minimised and the disc returned to storage medium as soon as possible.

3.10.3.2 Unfavourable Graft Profile from Manual Dissection

Preparation of the donor disc by manual lamellar dissection requires considerable skill and the potential exists for grafts to be produced which are too thick or with an uneven profile. A thick graft may induce a hypermetropic shift and may also crowd the iridocorneal angle, increasing the risk of glaucoma. A graft which is much thinner centrally than at the edge may act as a lenticule and also induce a hypermetropic shift. An asymmetric graft may induce astigmatism or higher-order aberrations, such as coma.

3.10.3.3 Endothelium Damage

The damage can happen during the implantation of the folding graft or inserting into the glide. Tissue handling must be delicate and minimal.

3.10.3.4 Inadequate Stripping of the Descemet's Membrane from the Host

If the Descemet's membrane is not removed over the whole area where the graft will attach, it may not attach well resulting in corneal oedema and poor vision (although some cases have been reported with successful outcomes without stripping at all).

3.10.3.5 Damage to the Lens (Phakic Patient)

Manoeuvring the graft into place in a phakic patient is difficult due to the restricted space, and damage may occur to the lens and/or the graft. Many surgeons prefer to remove the crystalline lens and allow the intraocular inflammation to settle before undertaking DSEK. Some surgeons undertake combined cataract extraction and DSEK as a triple procedure. This has the advantage of a single procedure, but IOL power prediction is difficult and the increased inflammation may compromise graft survival.

3.10.3.6 Excessive Intraocular Pressure from Air Bubble

After positioning the graft, the large air bubble placed in the anterior chamber raises the IOP substantially in order to tamponade it in place and aid adhesion. This may have adverse effects on the retinal vasculature (vascular occlusion) and optic nerve head and should be moderated in patients with advanced glaucoma.

3.10.3.7 Viscoelastic at Interface Preventing Graft Adhesion

Before inserting the graft, the viscoelastic should be removed from the anterior chamber completely to prevent it being retained at the graft-host interface as it will interfere with the graft adhesion. Dispersive viscoelastic substances should be avoided during DSEK because of the difficulty in ensuring complete removal by aspiration.

3.10.4 Postoperative Complications of PKP

3.10.4.1 Wound Leak

Leakage can be detected with Seidel's test and may be associated with flat or shallow anterior chamber. Small leaks may seal after placement of a bandage contact lens; larger leaks will require re-suturing.

3.10.4.2 Inflammation (Especially Paediatric Grafts)

Inflammation has to be controlled with topical steroids, the frequency adjusted according to the clinical response (Figs. 3.35 and 3.36). Uncontrolled inflammation is a risk factor for graft rejection (use of systemic steroids may be required).

3.10.4.3 Glaucoma

High intraocular pressure should initially be managed with topical medication but may require filtration surgery at a later stage.

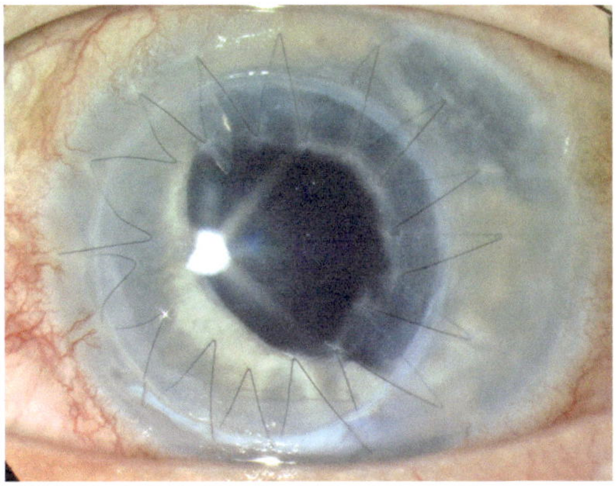

Fig. 3.35 Severe inflammation 1 month after PKP with loose suture at 8 o'clock

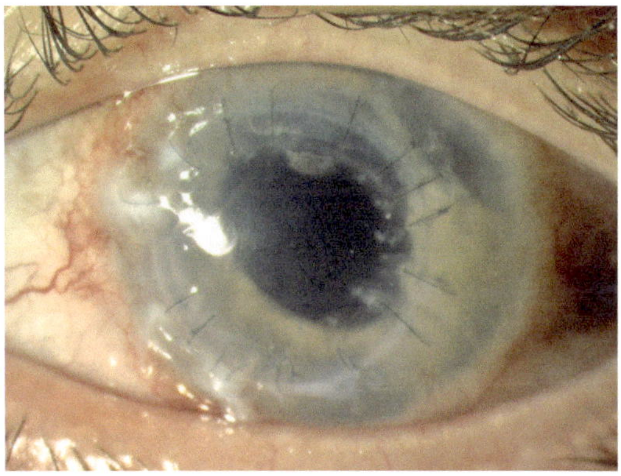

Fig. 3.36 Ongoing inflammation and suture replacement (same patient as Fig. 3.35)

3.10.4.4 Endothelial Graft Rejection

The most common type of graft rejection by far is endothelial rejection, followed by epithelial and stromal rejection. Endothelial rejections occur after at least a 2-week period of graft clarity; the mean onset for endothelial rejection is 8 months; late onset after, for example, 20 years is possible. Clinically, there is classically a distinct line demarcating the advancing immunological reaction (Khodadoust line). This is often pigmented and the area of cornea beyond which it has advanced is oedematous due to loss of endothelial cells. Treatment is with either intensive topical steroids (e.g. preservative-free dexamethasone 0.1 % hourly), supplemented with oral or pulsed intravenous methylprednisolone 500–1,000 mg (depending on body weight) daily for 3 days. The response is monitored by visual acuity, clinical examination and corneal thickness measurements. Rapid control of rejection episodes is desirable as the immune reaction destroys endothelial cells resulting in a reduced endothelial cell density. Repeated episodes of endothelial rejection may result in graft failure due to insufficient endothelial function to maintain graft dehydration and clarity. Graft rejection is mediated by T-cells. Specific T-cell inhibitors such as cyclosporin A and tacrolimus administered systemically have been shown to be useful as adjuncts to steroids in reducing the risk of rejection in high-risk cases and treating graft rejection in cases unresponsive to steroids.

3.10.4.5 Epithelial Graft Rejection

Epithelial rejections most frequently occur 1 month after keratoplasty; mean onset is 3 months; most are within the first year. Graft failure from this type of rejection is uncommon and relatively benign. Sometimes epithelial rejections forecast endothelial rejections. At the slit lamp a thin rejection line is seen in the corneal epithelium, starting in the periphery near the graft-host junction, migrating centrally over days, finally across the entire graft. This elevated line stains with fluorescein and rose bengal. There is minimal or no inflammation present. Primary treatment should be prompt with topical corticosteroids.

3.10.4.6 Stromal Graft Rejection

Stromal rejections are very uncommon but can lead to graft failure. Slit-lamp examination reveals a patchy deep stromal infiltrate in the graft with ocular inflammation and progressive vascularisation.

3.10.4.7 Graft Failure

Primary graft failure (1 % in PKP) leads to a cloudy/oedematous graft from day 1 and never clears. Corneas with secondary graft failure are initially healthy but become cloudy and thickened years later without evidence of active rejection (Fig. 3.37).

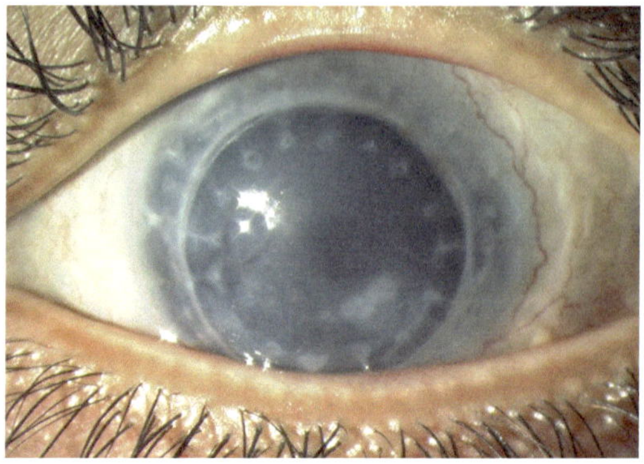

Fig. 3.37 Failed penetrating keratoplasty

3.10.4.8 Persistent Epithelial Defect

Restoration of an intact epithelium is a vital step in postoperative recovery as the graft is highly vulnerable to infection until this is achieved. If this is delayed beyond 1 week, damage to Bowman's layer can result in superficial haze; if coverage is delayed further, there may be stromal melting causing an uneven surface which impairs subsequent visual function. Transection of all the corneal nerves slows re-epithelialisation so the ocular surface environment must be optimised with tear supplements and lid hygiene measures as well as prophylactic antibiotics and control of inflammation. The surgeon should also consider punctal occlusion and bandage contact lenses to facilitate healing. In severe persistent epithelial defect, a tarsorrhaphy may be beneficial. Botulinum toxin can be given to the levator palpebrae superioris to induce ptosis for corneal protection, but the patient must understand that they must wait until new neuromuscular junctions are synthesised for the effect to wear off. This may take several months to resolve completely. The suggested dose is 5–10 units of Botox (Allergan Ltd, Marlow, UK) or 20 units of Dysport (Ipsen Ltd, Slough, UK); be aware of the dosage differences: 2.5 units of Dysport to equal 1 unit of Botox. The injection is with a 30G needle on an insulin syringe, aiming through the upper eyelid skin towards the orbital roof just inside the orbital rim.

3.10.4.9 Vascularisation of the Graft

If the graft becomes vascularised, it loses its immunological privilege and the risk of rejection is greatly increased. This can occur as a result of pre-existing inflammatory conditions (e.g. chemical injury, blepharitis, rheumatoid disease) or inflammation induced by the graft (e.g. microbial keratitis, loose suture trapping mucus). This can be reduced by optimising control of ocular surface inflammation preoperatively using topical lubricants and/or steroids, lid hygiene and even systemic immunosuppression if necessary. Postoperatively loose sutures must be removed once identified and corneal ulcers treated aggressively with intensive antibiotics or antiviral agents. If feeder vessels can be identified, it may be possible to treat them preoperatively with fine-needle micro-cautery or argon laser photocoagulation.

3.10.4.10 Suture-Related Complications

Loose or broken sutures (Fig. 1.10) should be removed as they contribute nothing to wound stability and are a focus for infection. If a continuous suture loosens very early (i.e. before sufficient would healing has occurred), it may be possible to restore adequate tension by placing a tensioning-loop suture in the host rim to loop through the continuous suture. If there is early loosening, the graft edge should be observed for slippage or dehiscence and re-sutured as necessary. Interrupted sutures which become vascularised should be considered for early removal to prevent vascularisation across the graft-host junction. Sutures with associated infiltrate (Fig. 1.11) should be removed taking care not to drag the infiltrate through the graft. Scarring of suture tracks is commonly seen in grafts (Fig. 3.38), especially in inflammatory eye disease, and is considered a minor complication.

3.10.4.11 Graft Dehiscence

A dehiscence of the graft may occur early, as a result of insufficient healing, or later, as a result of trauma. In older patients or those taking systemic steroids, the graft-host interface must be assessed carefully before suture removal is planned. If there is insufficient healing, it may be necessary to leave sutures indefinitely to prevent dehiscence. The graft-host interface will always be a weak point as the strength of the native cornea is never restored. Patients with penetrating keratoplasty should therefore be counselled to avoid contact sports or activities where trauma is likely and may be advised to wear polycarbonate safety glasses as routine.

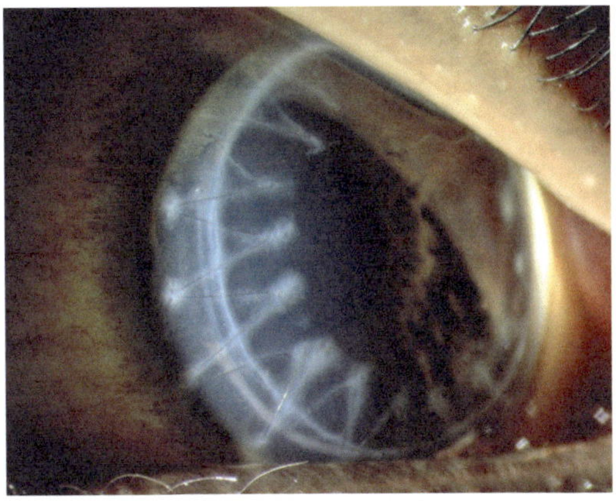

Fig. 3.38 Severe scarring of suture tracks 5 months after PKP

3.10.4.12 Corneal hypoaesthesia

Full-thickness trephination severs all corneal nerves so corneal sensation is reduced until there is re-growth. Restoration of sensation is an important step in achieving a healthy epithelium and the graft remains vulnerable to infection until this occurs. This may take some time and in some eyes is never achieved satisfactorily.

3.10.4.13 Dry Eye

This is exacerbated by inflammation and loss of corneal sensation and must be addressed with lid hygiene measures, tear supplements and/or punctum plugs as necessary.

3.10.4.14 Epithelial Down Growth

Proliferation of epithelium down into the interface and into the anterior chamber can cause secondary graft failure as the epithelium advances centripetally across the endothelium. This usually occurs within 3 months of penetrating keratoplasty and is a risk after wound dehiscence. It may also cause glaucoma, angle closure and inflammation. It may be difficult to distinguish between this and the classical pigmented rejection line seen in endothelial rejection and should be suspected if a presumed endothelial rejection does not respond to the steroid treatment.

3.10.4.15 Sterile Corneal Melt

This is a risk if epithelial healing is delayed or if there is chronic dry eye or poor control of inflammation. Immune mediators and proteolytic enzymes damage stromal collagen, causing irregularities in the corneal surface and risking subsequent secondary infection.

3.10.4.16 Corneal Astigmatism

Many factors contribute to post-keratoplasty astigmatism including poor surgical technique, mismatch in host/donor diameter and thickness, variable suture tension and orientation and uneven healing around the graft-host interface. Management of this is discussed below.

3.10.4.17 Cataract

Any procedure which disturbs the intraocular environment carries an increased risk of subsequent cataract formation, although this appears to be less with penetrating keratoplasty than with some other procedures. The lens is also vulnerable to direct trauma during the procedure which can be reduced by constricting the pupil preoperatively with topical pilocarpine 2 %.

3.10.4.18 Urrets-Zavalia Syndrome

This uncommon syndrome is characterised by a permanent atonic dilated pupil due to high intraocular pressure (also from air bubble) during and after surgery and presumed iris ischemia, especially in keratoconus patients. Treatment recommendations include a combination of sympatholytic and parasympathomimetic eye drops.

3.10.4.19 Infections

Small suture track infections (Fig. 1.11) are most common after penetrating keratoplasty and can be managed by removing an interrupted suture and prescribing frequent topical antibiotic.

The graft is also vulnerable to corneal ulcers due to reduced sensation and dry ocular surface. This must be treated aggressively as it is a major risk factor for rejection. The ulcer should be scraped for microbiological analysis and hourly broad-spectrum antibiotics prescribed. Admission to hospital for this should be considered.

Crystalline keratitis (Fig. 3.39) can be seen in eyes with long-term steroid treatment (such as in keratoplasty) and is suspicious for infection (Staphylococcus epidermidis, Streptococcus viridans and others). Treatment requires omission of steroids and start with topical antibiotics (e.g. ofloxacin).

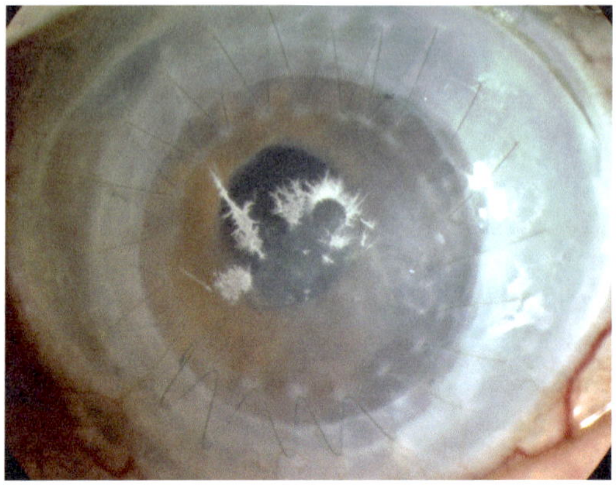

Fig. 3.39 Crystalline keratopathy in PKP

In rare cases (0.08–0.77 % of penetrating keratoplasty), a patient may develop postoperative endophthalmitis. The risk of this is increased if there is simultaneous cataract surgery and lens implantation, especially if an anterior vitrectomy is required. The risk can be reduced by giving intracameral or sub-conjunctival cefuroxime at the end of surgery. Presentation is usually within 72 h of surgery. If this is suspected, treatment should be aggressive with vitreous sampling, intravitreal and systemic antibiotics.

3.10.5 Postoperative Complications of DALK

Many of the complications that occur after penetrating keratoplasty can occur after DALK in a similar way, including glaucoma, inflammation, corneal hypoaesthesia, suture-related complications (Fig. 3.40), persistent epithelial defect and dry eye.

3.10.5.1 Double Anterior Chamber from Fluid/Viscoelastic at Interface

Micro-perforations in the Descemet's membrane during surgery can allow aqueous to leak postoperatively into the interface and prevent graft adhesion (Fig. 3.41). This is usually self-limiting and resolves in a few days. If the fluid collection is large, it may be necessary to inject a bubble of air

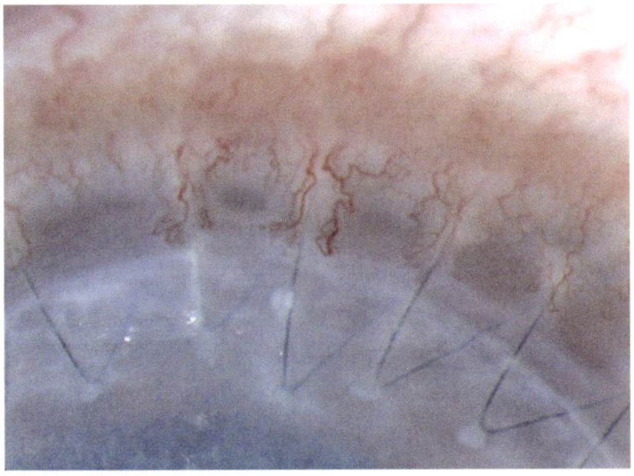

Fig. 3.40 Severe suture-related inflammation after DALK

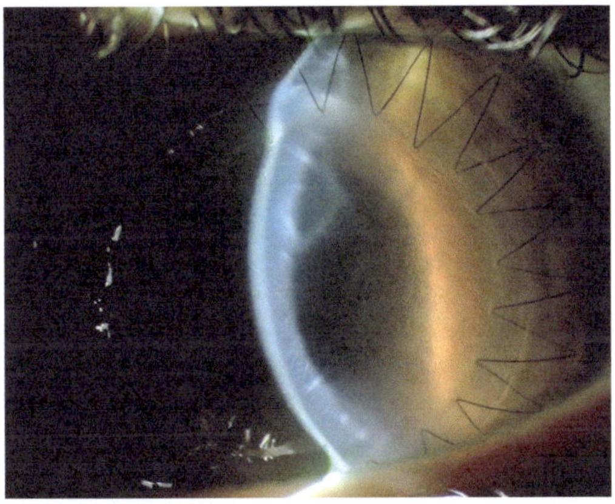

Fig. 3.41 Descemet's detachment after DALK

or expansile gas (e.g. SF_6) into the anterior chamber. Pupil block is a potential complication of this, and the risk can be reduced by keeping the pupil dilated and filling the anterior chamber no more than half-full of gas.

3.10.5.2 Folds in Graft Bed

Corneal folds are due to mechanical compression of the donor tissue and usually resolve over a few weeks postoperatively.

3.10.5.3 Interface Haze

If the host Descemet's membrane is not bared adequately, remaining stroma at the graft-host interface can lead to haze as the graft heals. Debris not removed by adequate irrigation will also remain at the interface and reduce graft clarity and visual quality.

3.10.5.4 Epithelial Down Growth

If the epithelium is incarcerated in the surgical wound before closure, epithelial proliferation along the graft-host interface can occur, reducing graft clarity.

3.10.5.5 Graft Rejection

Endothelial rejection is avoided as native endothelium remains in situ but epithelial or stromal rejection may still be seen, particularly if there is excessive inflammation or infection of the graft. Treatment may require penetrating keratoplasty.

3.10.5.6 Corneal Astigmatism

Astigmatism is generally less with DALK than with penetrating keratoplasty and can be addressed at an earlier stage postoperatively (see below).

3.10.6 Postoperative Complications of DSEK

3.10.6.1 Wrinkles in the Graft

The thin donor disc may form wrinkles as it attaches to host stroma. Attempts should be made at this stage to straighten these out by stroking the corneal surface with a smooth instrument, for example, Rycroft cannula or customised roller device. This may be easier while the anterior chamber is only partially filled with air. Postoperatively there is some scope for wrinkles to resolve, but major striae may be permanent and reduce visual quality.

3.10.6.2 Pupil Block Glaucoma

This can develop if the anterior chamber is left overfilled with air at the end of the procedure. The anterior chamber should only be left at the most half-filled with air so that aqueous is not prevented from flowing through the pupil and to the trabecular meshwork. If this is suspected, a small amount of air can be released via a paracentesis at the slit lamp.

3.10.6.3 Dislocated Graft

The most frequent early complication of DSEK is slippage of the graft (Figs. 3.42 and 3.43). This occurs when the patient sits up before

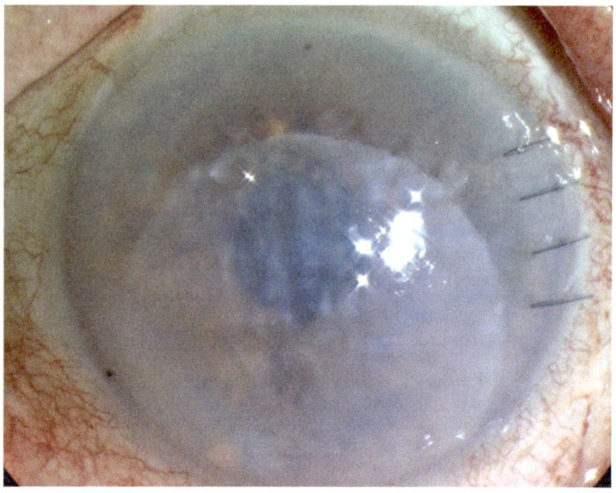

Fig. 3.42 Primary graft detachment after DSAEK (early, day 1)

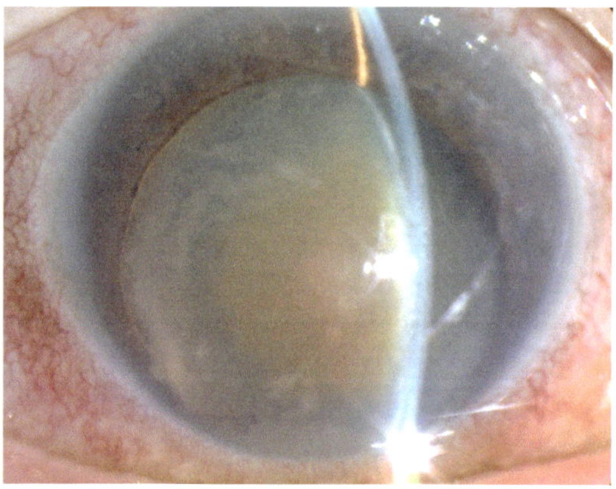

Fig. 3.43 Graft detachment after DSAEK (longstanding, 6 months, missed follow-ups)

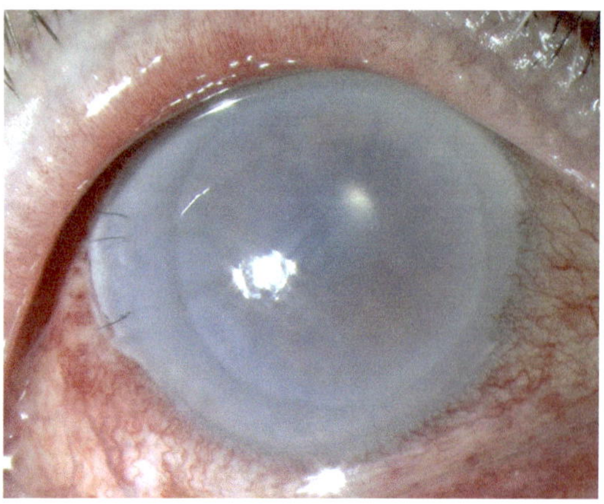

Fig. 3.44 Graft failure 10 weeks after DSAEK for Fuchs' endothelial dystrophy

adequate graft adhesion has occurred. It is therefore suggested that the patient remains supine while being transferred from the operating theatre to the preoperative unit/recovery area and remains supine for at least 2 h. The graft may be completely separated from the host or it may still be partially attached. The patient should return to theatre and the graft should be reattached. Air is injected into the anterior chamber via a paracentesis and the graft is positioned as during the original procedure. Further air tamponade and a longer period remaining supine usually allow secure attachment of the graft.

3.10.6.4 Graft Rejection

Endothelial rejection is possible but less common than in penetrating keratoplasty as there is less initial inflammation and topical steroid may be continued long term without the concern over impaired graft healing which is a limiting factor in the penetrating procedure. The patient must be monitored for secondary glaucoma, but if a low-potency agent such as fluorometholone is used, this is uncommon.

3.10.6.5 Graft Failure

Primary graft failure in DSAEK is about 10 to 30% following dislocation (Fig. 3.44). The manipulation involved in preparing the donor disc, and manoeuvring it into place means that there may be significant endothelial cell trauma. If this is excessive it may increase the primary failure rate, so great care must be taken throughout. It has been shown however that with care, endothelial cell loss at 1 year is comparable to after penetrating keratoplasty (Table 3.10).

3.10.7 Management of Corneal Astigmatism

Visual rehabilitation after keratoplasty is aimed at restoring optical clarity of the cornea and managing ametropia. Significant astigmatism is often seen, especially after penetrating keratoplasty (Fig. 3.45), and if this is irregular it may create challenges in restoration of useful vision. It is reasonable to assess this 3–6 months after surgery as

Table 3.10 Graft rejection rat, endothelial cell loss and post-keratoplasty refraction

	PKP	DALK	DSEK
Rejection episodes	15–25 % (1/5 irreversible)	10–15 %	5–8 % (1/3 asymptomatic)
Endothelial cell loss			
Over 1 year	15–37 %		30 %
Over 5 years	60 %		40 %
Mean postoperative astigmatism	4–5 D	4–5 D	1–2 D
Mean postoperative SE	−1.5 D	−4 D	

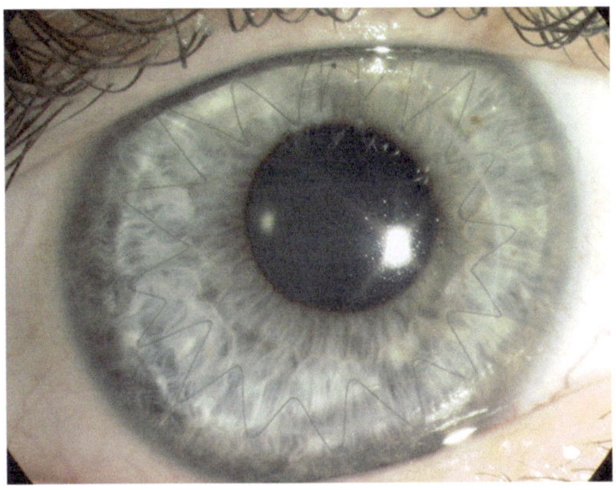

Fig. 3.45 5 D corneal astigmatism after PKP from irregular suturing (trainee surgeon)

early fluctuations in corneal morphology should have settled by this time. The patient is assessed with refraction, and topography and spectacles may be prescribed if the astigmatism is regular and low and there is little anisometropia. The patient must be aware that the spectacle refraction is likely to change over the next months, and especially after removal of the corneal sutures 12–18 months after surgery.

3.10.7.1 Suture Adjustment

If a continuous suture has been used, suture adjustment within the first 6 weeks may be used to reduce excessive corneal astigmatism. Adjustment beyond this time is of little use since healing at the graft-host interface creates rigidity which limits the effect of adjusting suture tension on corneal shape. Suture adjustment is ideally carried out under the operating microscope under guidance of the keratoscope. The suture should be freed up along its length, and loops are tightened at the flat meridians and loosened at the steep meridians. Care must be exercised not to break the suture – if this happens re-suturing is required. It may be possible to splice in a length of suture material and redo a few passes to assist with this and avoid replacing the entire suture.

If interrupted sutures have been used, they can be removed selectively according to the refraction and topography. One or more sutures at the steep meridian can be removed at the slit lamp with topical antibiotic and steroid cover. The disadvantage of this is that many such interventions may be required to address the astigmatism adequately and ultimately there may be no advantage in visual recovery over waiting and removing all the sutures at one later date.

3.10.7.2 Spectacles and Contact Lenses

Once all the sutures have been removed, the topography is likely to stabilise and a more reliable assessment can be made. If the astigmatism is regular, spectacles may be the least complex way to correct ametropia. Small amounts of irregular astigmatism may be addressed with rigid contact lenses. However, some patients are unable to tolerate this and request further surgical intervention. Large amounts of astigmatism may be correctable with glasses or contact lenses, but this may induce significant distortion, and the corrected vision may not be very useful in functional terms.

3.10.7.3 Arcuate Keratotomies

Arcuate keratotomy (AK) is useful for reducing large amounts of regular astigmatism (Fig. 3.46) or in combination with subsequent excimer laser for large amounts of irregular astigmatism. It corrects up to 4 D, and if more is required it can be combined with orthogonal compression sutures to 'hold the incisions open' and boost their effect. The arcuate incisions can be cut with precision depth-guided blade or the Femtosecond laser. Generally, the depth of the cut should be guided

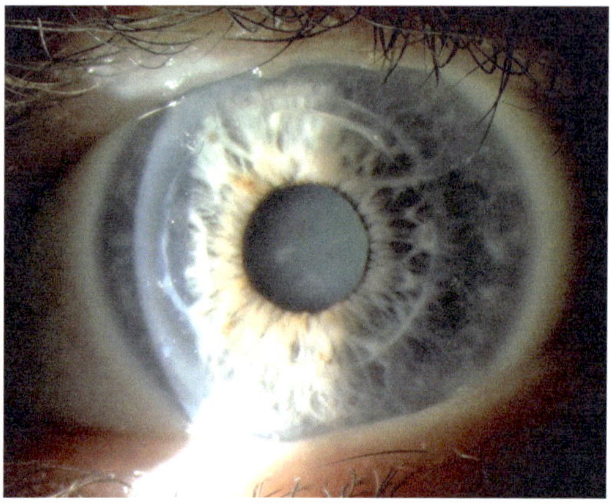

Fig. 3.46 Arcuate keratotomies for corneal astigmatism after PKP (from 5 to 2 D)

by pachymetry, for example, using the Visante pachymetry map which gives corneal thickness at various locations; aim for ≥95 % depth. Leaving deeper tissue uncut drastically reduces the effectiveness of the incision. The axis is marked with patients sitting to avoid errors induced by cyclotorsion. Incisions are mostly done inside the graft-host interface, but some surgeons perform more limbal located incisions. The use of AK nomograms can increase predictability, but there is still some unpredictability due to variation in healing and inherent compliance of the cornea. Check the change in astigmatism with an on-table keratoscope. If the effect is insufficient, try irrigating within the incision to further expand the gap. The incisions can trigger stromal melt in patients with dry eyes. Finally, prescribe topical antibiotic and steroid to avoid infection and rejection.

3.10.7.4 Excimer Laser

This technique is good for up to 6 D of corneal regular or irregular astigmatism. It can be combined with AKs to treat astigmatism over 6 D, and it simultaneously corrects myopia or hypermetropia. Laser ablation requires sufficient corneal thickness to leave an adequate residual stromal bed after ablation of approximately 300 μm. The preferred technical approach is LASEK in combination with mitomycin, which avoids flap-related complications such as displacement, melt or diffuse lamellar keratitis. It is also safer for thinner corneas and less likely to provoke dry eye as fewer corneal nerves are damaged. If LASIK is performed, it should be as a two-stage procedure, for example, the flap is cut and replaced in a first stage, followed by topography and eventually wavefront scans to analyse the refractive change of flap creation. In a second procedure, the flap is then lifted and the ablation profile applied. Uneven tension in the graft-host interface may make healing of the flap unpredictable and give unpredictable refractive outcomes. When the flap is cut and lifted, this may release some of the tension, and the forces acting on the stromal bed are altered, potentially leading to an inappropriate treatment being applied. For LASEK and LASIK, a bandage contact lens should be placed at the end of the procedure. The patient should be prescribed topical preservative-free antibiotic, steroid and tear supplements and monitored closely for recovery of epithelium and signs of infection and dry eye.

3.10.7.5 Toric Intraocular Lens Implantation

Different types of toric intraocular lenses (IOL) can be used to correct regular (and possibly also irregular) corneal astigmatism in phakic patients. The Verisyse, Artisan or Artiflex iris clip lenses, for example, are designed for phakic patients and can be implanted via small incision. Patients with minimal cataract may benefit from clear lens extraction with implantation of a toric IOL in the capsular bag. Models of this type of lenses include AcrySof SN60TT toric IOL and Rayner T-Flex lenses (Fig. 3.47). Customised toric IOLs are suitable for correcting larger amounts of regular astigmatism, myopia and hypermetropia in eyes after PKP, DALK and DSEK. At the beginning of the procedure, horizontal zero-degree reference marks are placed at the slit lamp. The toric IOLs are then inserted through a scleral tunnel or limbal corneal incision to minimise induced astigmatism. Extra care should be taken not to further compromise the endothelium and to minimise postoperative inflammation. Phakic patients undergoing iris clip IOL implantation should have endothelial cell density (ECD) and anterior chamber characteristics measured preoperatively (e.g. with OCT or Pentacam) to ensure safety. ECD should be assessed annually after surgery. Smaller amounts of refractive errors in pseudophakic keratoplasty patients can be corrected with the implantation of a sulcus-fixated supplementary intraocular lens (e.g. Rayner Sulcoflex aspheric or toric; Fig. 3.48).

Table 3.11 summarises common approaches to correct astigmatism after keratoplasty.

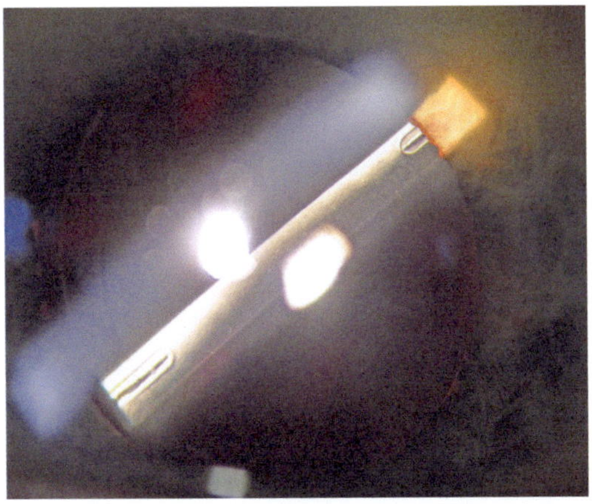

Fig. 3.47 Toric intraocular lens at 40° (Rayner T-Flex)

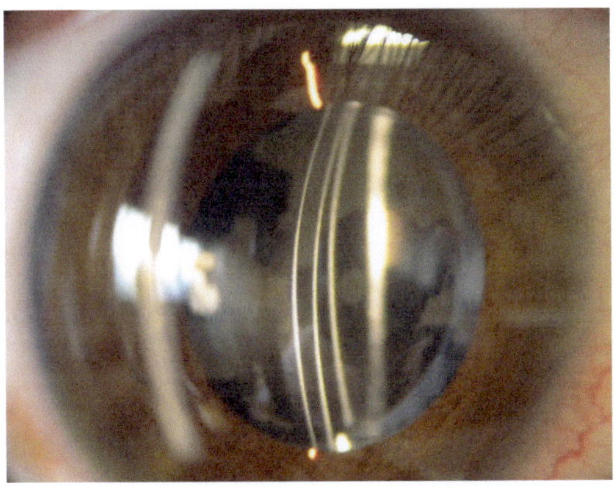

Fig. 3.48 Supplementary toric intraocular lens (Rayner Sulcoflex Toric)

Table 3.11 Approaches to correct post-keratoplasty astigmatism

	High astigmatism	Low astigmatism
Regular	AK + compression sutures	AK
	AK then toric IOL or LASEK	LASEK/LASIK Toric IOL
Irregular	Arcuate keratotomy then LASEK	LASEK/LASIK

3.11 Outcomes of Keratoplasty

3.11.1 Graft Survival

Survival of the graft refers to maintenance of an optically clear cornea with no signs of oedema from endothelial decompensation. Graft failure can be primary (graft never clears after transplant), delayed primary (clear for more than 2 weeks and then becomes cloudy and oedematous in the absence of rejection) or secondary (usually due to allograft rejection). National corneal graft registries record data regarding graft function, rejection episodes and additional procedures at various time points after transplant. This has generated huge datasets which have contributed to better understanding of the process and dynamic of graft rejection and failure.

The graft survival is influenced by a number of factors including:

- Patient behaviour, such as compliance with topical medication and careful hand hygiene, can reduce the risk of infection and rejection. Graft failure and rejection are both more common in younger patients: the risk of rejection and failure is twice as likely in patients under 40 years. In children younger than 15 years, the graft survival rate is as low as 60–70 % at 2 years for first-time grafts.
- Recipient beds for transplants with no history of ocular inflammation (e.g. keratoconus) are associated with better survival than those with previous inflammation or vascularisation (e.g. HSK). Transplants made into an eye with active inflammation (e.g. emergency graft for an inflammatory melt/perforation) have an even poorer prognosis. Peripheral anterior synechiae are associated with a higher failure risk.
- Careful surgical technique maximises endothelial cell survival and is associated with longer graft survival.
- Correct postoperative management of complications reduces the chance of early graft failure. Glaucoma is associated with poorer graft survival and must be managed adequately.
- Time factor: corneal transplants have a limited lifespan and even in uncomplicated cases may

fail eventually due to chronic endothelial cell attrition (Figs. 3.49 and 3.50). If multiple grafts are required over time, every new graft has a higher failure rate.

Risk of failure can be assessed preoperatively (Table 3.12), and the graft survival rate for primary keratoplasties depends on the procedure and indication, as data from the UK corneal transplant registry 2010 showed (Table 3.13).

For high-risk grafts, the heterogeneous nature of conditions and difficulty in both stratifying risk and defining 'high risk' make it difficult to assign patients to different levels of risk. This also makes it difficult for a clinician to estimate the likelihood of graft survival. However, for certain high-risk grafts, rates of rejection can be up to 70 % despite topical and systemic immunosuppressant medication.

3.11.2 Refractive Outcomes

After DALK, astigmatism typically ranges between 3.0 and 5.0 D. Astigmatism tends to be slightly higher after PKP and more irregular; but overall there is not much difference between these two groups. Many suture techniques have been proposed to reduce induced astigmatism (including interrupted, continuous, double torque/anti-torque continuous and combined interrupted and continuous), but there seems little difference in the final outcome. Grafts cut with the femtosecond laser can be made to fit very closely with a complementary profile cut in the host rim, and these heal securely with fewer and less tight sutures. It may be that this induces less astigmatism and allows faster healing and earlier removal of sutures.

The spherical equivalent of the grafted eye will depend on a number of factors including preoperative refractive error, keratometry of the donor cornea, donor and host size, suture technique (type of suture and tension) and any intra- or postoperative complication. For example, tight sutures may result in flatter corneal curvature and induce hypermetropia.

There is often a small hyperopic shift (around +1 D) after DSEK, but some series have reported that on average, the procedure is refractive neutral.

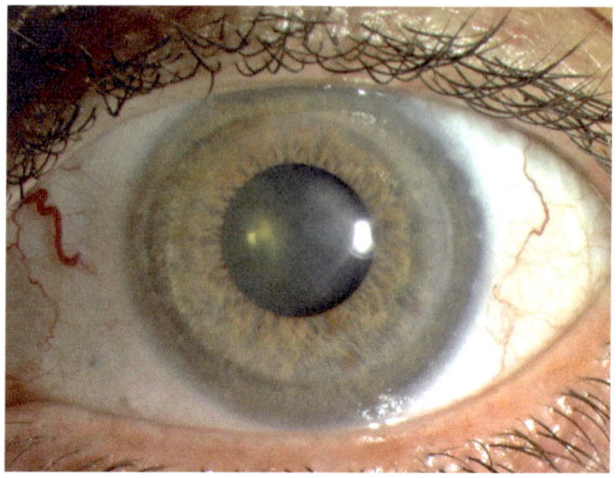

Fig. 3.49 Long-term success: clear cornea 20 years after PKP for keratoconus

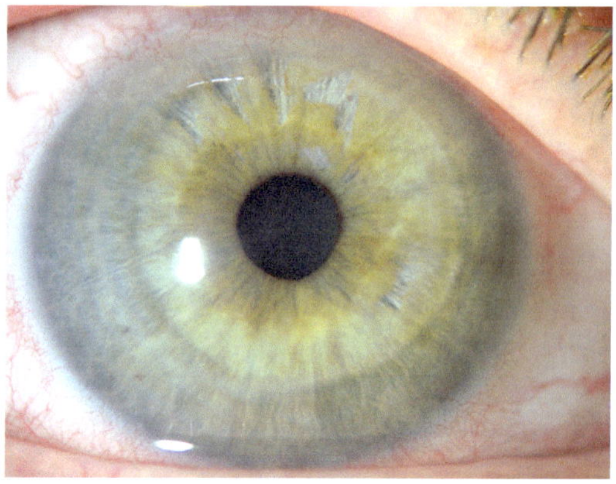

Fig. 3.50 Long-term success: clear cornea 18 years after PKP for keratoconus

3.11.3 Visual Outcomes

After PKP and DALK, visual rehabilitation is slow and patients should be counselled that it may take 1–2 years for them to achieve their best vision. Visual acuity can be expected to improve slowly over this time. Recovery tends to be quicker after DALK than PKP with less astigmatism. Subjective refraction should be performed around 3 months post-op and contact lenses or glasses prescribed if appropriate to maximise visual function. The prescription is liable to change, and this can be repeated every 4 months or after selective suture removal.

Specifically for patients undergoing keratoplasty for keratoconus, a corrected distance visual acuity (CDVA) of 6/6 or better is more likely at 1, 2 and 4 years post-op after PKP than after DALK (lamellar dissection). On average one Snellen

Table 3.12 Risk of failure of keratoplasty

Low risk (90 % success)	Medium risk (50–80 % success)	High risk (>50 % success)
First transplant	Repeat grafts	Active inflammation (OCP)
Non-inflammatory	Previous corneal inflammation	Emergency graft
No active surface disease	Corneal neovascularisation	Limbal stem cell deficiency
No corneal neovascularisation	Advanced Fuchs' ED	Previous graft failure
Keratoconus	Herpetic eye disease	Severe chemical injuries
Early Fuchs' ED	Young children	Congenial glaucoma
Lattice dystrophy	Macular dystrophy	Advanced dry eye syndrome
Corneal scars (non-herpetic)	Rheumatoid arthritis	Children
	CHED	

Table 3.13 Graft survival rate for primary keratoplasties

Time	PKP	DALK	DSEK
1 year	Keratoconus: 97 % Fuchs' ED: 97 % All indications: 93 %	Keratoconus: 97 %	Fuchs' ED: 90 %
2 years	Keratoconus: 95 % Fuchs' ED: 93 % All indications: 87 %	Keratoconus: 94 %	Fuchs' ED: 72 %
5 years (2011)	Keratoconus: 92 %	Keratoconus: 90 %	
10 years	Keratoconus: >90 % Fuchs' ED: 60 % HSV inactive: 45 % PBK: 30 %	Keratoconus: >80 %	

line of acuity difference is to be expected between these groups. CDVA after DALK by lamellar dissection may be limited by uneven recipient dissection, interface haze or particulate debris trapped at the interface which may cause light scatter and haze. For DALK, some studies report better CDVA outcomes with the big-bubble technique suggesting that interface haze is a limiting factor and the smoother the interface can be made, the better. A recent study of patients undergoing keratoplasty for various pathologies found that visual acuity and refractive outcomes at 1 year were comparable between PKP and DALK (big-bubble technique) cohorts (Table 3.14).

Table 3.14 Visual outcomes in keratoplasty

	PKP	DALK	DSEK
Mean CDVA	6/6 (20/20)	6/7.5 (20/25)	6/7.5 (20/25)
Mean CDVA ≥ 6/12 (20/40)	Keratoconus: 90 % Fuchs' ED: 50 % PBK: 20 %	90 %	90 %
Mean CDVA >6/6 (20/20) or better after 5 years	39 %	29 %	

Patients requiring unilateral keratoplasty (PKP or DALK) who have a healthy fellow eye should be aware that image quality in the grafted eye will probably never match that of the un-operated eye, even if post-keratoplasty ametropia is addressed aggressively. This is probably due to a greater amount of higher-order aberrations induced by the keratoplasty.

Visual recovery after DSEK (and especially DMEK) is much faster and patients can expect an improvement in the first few months after surgery (even sooner after DMEK). Visual acuity is slightly better at 1 month post-op after than DSAEK than after DSEK, but there is no difference by 3 months. After DSEK/DSAEK the CDVA is usually slightly limited by interface haze, but this generally fades over the 12–24 months following surgery. However, if there has been severe or chronic stromal oedema preoperatively, permanent structural changes may have occurred in the host stroma which then limit potential CDVA. As the safety of surgery increases, it may become advantageous to offer endothelial replacement earlier rather than later.

Interestingly, some patients whose measured Snellen acuity does not seem to have improved substantially after DSEK for Fuchs' endothelial dystrophy (Fuchs' ED) report a subjective improvement with which they are quite happy. It is possible that the diseased endothelium induces scatter which degrades the image quality more than reducing acuity; addressing this may improve perceived image quality more than resolution.

As early as 1–3 months after DMEK, around 90 % of patients with no ocular co-morbidity recover CDVA of 6/12 (20/20) or better, and 60 % have a CDVA of 6/9 (20/32) or better. At 6 months these figures were 95 and 75 %, respectively. A hyperopic shift of around 0.5 D can be expected, with little or no change in astigmatism.

Refractive Corneal Surgery

4

4.1 Incisional Corneal Surgery

Incisional techniques for reducing corneal astigmatism are based on Gauss' law of inelastic domes. A circumferential arcuate incision made on the steep corneal axis will cause slight flattening of that axis coupled with a corresponding steepening of the orthogonal axis. The spherical equivalent of the cornea usually remains essentially unchanged (coupling ratio = 1). However, in very long or very short incisions, the amounts of flattening and steepening differ. For arcuate incisions <20°, there is more flattening, causing a hyperopic shift. The reverse applies to long incisions (>90°).

Incisions can be made at the limbus (e.g. in conjunction with cataract surgery when addressing high corneal astigmatism) or in clear cornea. After penetrating keratoplasty or deep anterior lamellar keratoplasty, the incisions can be made at the graft-host junction or just inside the interface. Incisions can be made with a guarded depth blade or the femtosecond laser. Blades can be preset to a specific depth or may be micrometre adjustable. A diamond blade with a single footplate gives good visualisation of the incision depth and angle. An alternative is to use an astigmatome, a device like a trephine which fits into a vacuum ring secured to the globe. The protruding blades on the astigmatome create the incision as the device is rotated through the desired angle.

Such circumferential incisions can be typically used to correct up to 3 D (dioptres) of astigmatism. Nomograms can be used to determine the number, length and depth of incision and must take into account preoperative keratometry, corneal diameter and patient age. Paired incisions are usually favoured to reduce the risk of inducing irregular astigmatism. With sufficient experience and consistency of instruments, a surgeon may choose to customise his nomogram, based on his own refractive outcomes.

4.1.1 Radial Keratotomy

Radial keratotomy (RK) was one of the early refractive surgical procedures and was developed during the 1960s to correct myopia up to 8 D. Using a very sharp diamond blade, deep radial stromal incisions were placed in the mid-periphery of the cornea (Fig. 4.1). The effect of this was to

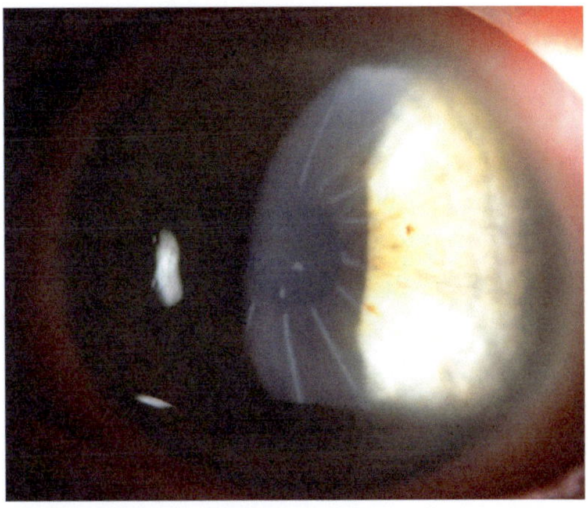

Fig. 4.1 Radial keratotomy

B. Zuberbuhler et al., *Corneal Surgery*,
DOI 10.1007/978-3-642-12502-7_4, © Springer-Verlag Berlin Heidelberg 2013

weaken the mid-periphery and allow the cornea to bulge, thus steepening the mid-periphery and flattening the corneal apex. The blade had a special footplate which allowed the surgeon to place four, six or eight incisions set at 100% depth of the thinnest of four paracentral ultrasound pachymetry measurements. A central optical zone of 3 or 4 mm was spared and the incisions were extended to the limbus peripherally.

The procedure was effective at correcting myopia but had an unacceptably low predictability and a high complication rate. Complications included glare, infection and melting, and the incisions weakened the globe integrity to the extent that rupture with minor trauma was common even many years later and these eyes were put at high risk of subsequently developing ectasia.

The Prospective Evaluation of Radial Keratotomy (PERK) study found that at 10 years after surgery 53 % of eyes had uncorrected visual acuities of 6/6 or better and 85 % saw 6/12 or better uncorrected. However, it also found that the 90 % prediction interval was >4 D wide and that between 6 months and 10 years after surgery, 43 % of eyes experienced a hyperopic shift of ≥1 D. The degree of hyperopic shift was greater when a smaller clear central optical zone was used. In addition to this, a subset of the cohort had residual refractive errors which fluctuated in a clear diurnal pattern. No patient factors were observed to be consistently associated with refractive unpredictability.

For these reasons of unpredictability and long-term instability, RK has become obsolete and has been replaced by excimer laser refractive corrections and intraocular lens implants (ICL, ACIOL or iris clip types).

Excimer laser refractive surgery is also an option for post-RK refractive errors, although debate exists over whether LASEK or LASIK should be the procedure of choice. Both appear to be safe and effective.

For correction of ectasia, PKP may be needed. This may be technically difficult due to the presence of deep radial scars and may incur problems postoperatively associated with crossing corneal incisions and the subsequent increased risk of melting. A cohort of 16 patients (24 eyes) who had had previous RK for keratoconus and who subsequently underwent PKP attained mean BSCVA of 6/9 at last follow-up with a mean of 3.6 D of corneal astigmatism. Episodes of graft rejection were seen in six eyes, but only one required a regraft. Corneal collagen cross-linking has also been reported to be safe and effective for treatment of ectasia after RK, but experience with this is still limited.

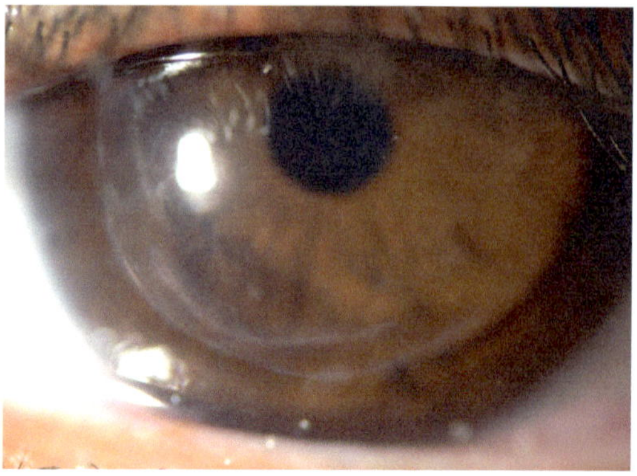

Fig. 4.2 Arcuate keratotomy in the corneal transplant

4.1.2 Arcuate Keratotomy

Arcuate keratotomies (AK) have greater effect when placed closer to the visual axis (more centrally) and are usually placed around a 6–8 mm optical zone. Incisions within the 6 mm optical zone should be avoided because they result in irregular astigmatism and may cause glare (Fig. 4.2). A second pair of incisions may be placed to enhance the effect of the first by 25–33 %. However, there is no benefit from placing more than two pairs. In eyes with previous radial keratotomy, the surgeon must take care that radial and arcuate incisions do not cross, which would lead to poor tissue healing and ectasia with poor visual results.

4.1.2.1 Preparation

Preoperative topography must demonstrate stable corneal astigmatism. Topical anaesthetic is given and the positions of 3 and 9 o'clock meridia marked with ink on the cornea with the patient sitting. This can be done freehand or there are a range of alignment devices for use with the slit lamp. This is to account for cyclotorsion when the patient lies supine.

4.1.2.2 Technique

The procedure is carried out under topical anaesthesia under the microscope with a speculum in place. The landmarks identified preoperatively guide placement of axis marker instruments (e.g. Mendez degree gauge or Zuberbuhler toric marker) which allow the steep axis and the extent of the incision to be marked. A guarded blade set to 95–100 % of the central corneal thickness is used to make the incisions and held so that the incision is made perpendicular to the corneal surface. The surgeon must press firmly to ensure adequate depth of incision as shallow incisions will be ineffective. It is usually easier and a more controlled action to pull the blade towards oneself while cutting than to push it away. The result is assessed with on-table keratoscopy. If the effect is insufficient, the incisions can be opened with a Rycroft cannula and irrigated with BSS for a slightly enhanced effect (also washes out epithelial cells).

4.1.2.3 Aftercare

Postoperatively topical antibiotic and lubricant are given. If the patient has had a corneal graft, topical steroid is also given to reduce the chance of rejection. Close follow-up is needed especially for patients with dry eyes because of the risk of triggering a corneal melt.

4.1.2.4 Enhancements

The refractive effect can be enhanced by placing 9/0 nylon compression sutures at 90° from the arcuate incisions. These should stay in place for 12 weeks (or longer) before assessing the refractive outcome. If there is overcorrection, the compression sutures can be removed. If the outcome is acceptable, the sutures may remain in place longer.

4.1.3 Ruiz Procedure

Also known as trapezoidal keratotomy, this technique combines paired arcuate incisions with radial keratotomies ('corridor incisions') and was intended to flatten the steep meridian while having little or no effect on the orthogonal meridian (90° away). In the original description, the tangential and radial incisions connected, but this was associated with melting and ectasia. This was later modified so that the incisions did not meet up to avoid these complications. Terry and Rowsey showed in 1986 that this procedure was able to alter corneal astigmatism by up to 11 D in cadaver eyes. Results in vivo have been very variable however and its unpredictability has meant that this operation has fallen out of favour in some circles. Other complications, including monocular diplopia and glare, have also been reported.

4.1.4 Limbal Relaxing Incisions

Partial-thickness incisions placed near the limbus to correct astigmatism have a long heritage and predate Zirm's first successful human corneal transplant. Limbal relaxing incisions (LRIs) can be used combined with cataract surgery, after penetrating keratoplasty or deep anterior lamellar keratoplasty, to correct small amounts of regular astigmatism (up to 3.5 D) or to reduce a large astigmatic error to a magnitude which can then be corrected by excimer laser refractive surgery.

The principle is the same as for arcuate keratotomies in that an incision on the meridian of steepest corneal curvature results in flattening of that meridian, coupled with steepening of the meridian 90° away.

Compared with AK, LRIs are more forgiving and require less accurate placement. They are also less likely to induce either a change in axis or irregular astigmatism. They are technically easier to perform and the coupling effect is more predictable. They tend to cause little discomfort and the incisions usually heal well without causing much dry eye syndrome. The disadvantage is that a longer arc length is required to achieve the same refractive effect compared to AKs.

The procedure is similar to that described above for AKs, but the incisions are placed in the most peripheral clear cornea, just inside the surgical limbus. A blade set to 90 % of the thinnest pachymetry reading at the limbus can be used, or alternatively, a standard 600 μm blade is usually appropriate. Any bleeding from pannus can be ignored as it will stop spontaneously.

4.1.5 Complications of Arcuate or Limbal Relaxing Incisions

Potential complications include infection, full-thickness incision (which requires suturing as the incision will not self-seal), wound gape, under- or overcorrection, misalignment, induced irregular astigmatism, decreased corneal sensation and reduced globe strength.

4.2 Corneal Implants

4.2.1 Introduction

Intrastromal ring segments were initially designed for correcting low to moderate myopia, but the results were rather imprecise and the introduction of excimer laser correction of myopia with its high level of precision soon afterwards relegated this application to the annals of history. There has been a resurgence of interest however in the use of intrastromal rings in the management of corneal ectatic disorders, particularly keratoconus and pellucid marginal degeneration. The effect on the more pliable tissue in these disorders is greater than that seen in 'normal' corneal tissue in the treatment of myopia. There may also be a role in the management of post-refractive surgery ectasia.

All ring segments are made of transparent PMMA of precise dimensions which are inserted into the mid-peripheral corneal stroma. The principle is that the corneal periphery is thickened, leading to a flattening of the central cornea. The amount of flattening is inversely proportional to the diameter of the ring segments. The ring segments also ensure that the deformation forces (due to intraocular pressure) acting on the cornea are applied more evenly, reducing the tendency of the cornea to 'bulge' in areas of thinning and weakness. This reduces the overall tendency of the refractive error of keratoconus to progress.

The clinical objectives in intrastromal ring segment implantation are:

- To reduce corneal irregularity so that contact lens fitting is easier
- To reduce corneal irregularity in conjunction with collagen cross-linking
- To correct myopia
- To avoid the need for penetrating or deep anterior lamellar keratoplasty

4.2.2 Types of Implants

There are three main types of intrastromal corneal ring segments:

4.2.2.1 Intacs (Addition Technology Inc.)

Intacs are patented hexagonal and oval ring segments and are placed outside the 5 mm optical zone. These rings are FDA and NICE approved as safe and effective for keratoconus (NICE Guidance IPG 227). The refractive effect is modulated by the Intacs' thickness. Intacs segments are available in thicknesses from 210 to 450 μm and the implant should be chosen according to the manifest refractive error (sphere and cylinder) and corneal topography. A nomogram is available for guiding implant choice.

4.2.2.2 Ferrara Rings (Ferrara Ophthalmics)

In contrast to Intacs, these rings are triangular in profile (cross section) and are placed just inside a 5 mm optical zone, chosen according to degree of myopia, symmetry of cone and stage of keratoconus. The triangular profile of these segments was chosen to reduce dysphotopsia such as haloes. The depth of the pocket is 80 % of (central) corneal thickness. Ferrara rings are available in two diameters/optical zones: 5 mm optical zone (inner and outer diameters are 4.4 and 5.4 mm) and 6 mm optical zone (5.4 and 6.4 mm diameters). In mixed, irregular or hyperopic astigmatism, a single ring segment can be used.

Table 4.1 Visual outcomes in keratoplasty

	Intacs			
	Standard	SK	Ferrara rings	Kerarings
Arc length (°)	150	150	90–210	90–210
Cross section	Hexagonal	Oval	Triangular	Triangular
Thickness (μm)	250–450	400 and 450	150–350	150–350
Radius of curvature:				
Inner (mm)	6.77	6	4.4 and 5.4	4.4–5.4
Outer (mm)	8.10	7.4	5.6 and 6.4	5.6–6.4

4.2.2.3 Kerarings (Mediphacos)

The Keraring and Ferrara ring are very similar in design, shape and size. Both systems are versatile, offering 40 combinations of ring segment thicknesses (segment's effect), arc lengths (modulation of sphere and cylinder correction) and optical zones (addressing variations in pachymetry and stages of disease). Kerarings are available with optical zones of 5, 5.5 and 6 mm and should be implanted at 75 % corneal depth. Depending on the case, one or two Keraring segments of the same or different sizes may be implanted. Nomograms are available from the manufacturer.

Basic characteristics of different ring segments are shown in Table 4.1.

4.2.3 Technique

Preoperative planning must include recent topography and pachymetry across a number of locations on the cornea, particularly in the regions where the tunnels will be placed. A Visante OCT (Carl Zeiss Meditec) or Pentacam pachymetry map is ideal for this.

The main advantages of intrastromal ring implantation are that it is relatively non-invasive, short procedure and performed under local anaesthetic. It is reversible and the rings are easily removed if necessary. The main disadvantage is that the refractive outcomes are still somewhat unpredictable.

Options for placement of ring segments:

- Place on steeper axis to reduce astigmatism with rings centred on the visual axis
- Place so that the centre of the rings is aligned with the centre of the cone (i.e. decentred from the geometric centre of the cornea by up to 1.5 mm)

The intrastromal tunnels for the ring segment placement can be dissected mechanically with a rotating blade or with the femtosecond laser.

4.2.3.1 Mechanical Tunnel Creation

The pupil centre or visual axis is marked as desired and an inked template is used to mark the cornea to guide where the rings will lie and where the incision should be made. The incision should be 1 mm from the limbus and is usually temporal, so that the rings will lie above and below the marked centre. A radial incision 1mm long is made with a guarded diamond blade to 70 % depth of the corneal thickness of the flattest topographical axis. A pocketing knife is then inserted into the incision and used to initiate the tunnels. The vacuum ring is then applied ensuring careful alignment and the tunnel creators are rotated within this guide to create the tunnels in clockwise and anticlockwise directions. The intrastromal ring is rinsed in sterile preservative-free chloramphenicol (Minims), grasped with the special forceps and introduced into the tunnel. The initial incision is sutured with 10/0 nylon; further topical antibiotic can be given. A bandage contact lens may be used.

Mechanical tunnel formation carries the risks of epithelial defects, perforations (anterior and posterior), extension of the incision towards the visual axis or the limbus, shallow or uneven placement of ring segments, epithelial ingrowth, introduction of infection via the blade, decentration, stromal thinning and stromal oedema around the incision and channel.

4.2.3.2 Tunnel Creation with the Femtosecond Laser

The procedure is largely similar. The cornea is marked for the desired centration of the rings and the laser programmed for tunnel depth and arc location. The vacuum ring is applied and the laser is docked with the patient's eye. Once the tunnels are created, the rings can be inserted as above. The incision rarely requires suturing. Topical antibiotic is given.

The use of a femtosecond laser gives slightly better results for patients with keratoconus, as the tunnels can be placed with more precision and less tissue manipulation. Care must still be taken to ensure accurate centration as there may be asymmetric flattening of the cornea during the applanation process and the pupil may dilate eccentrically. A further advantage of femtosecond laser tunnel creation is reduced risk of infection (as no blade is introduced into the tunnel), lower risk of epithelial defect and less stromal oedema. The more precise incision rarely requires suturing. Deposits are sometimes seen in the lamellar channel alongside the rings. These probably include lipid and extracellular debris from keratocytes activated during the initial wound-healing response. It is suggested that femtosecond laser created tunnels, being smaller and having less space around the implant, would have a lower tendency to show these deposits.

4.2.3.3 Postoperative Management

Topical antibiotic and steroid are given and tapered according to the observed response (e.g. G chloramphenicol preservative-free qds 1 month and G dexamethasone qds 1 month tapering over the next 2 months to zero). Careful attention is paid to healing of the incision and any signs of inflammation or infection in the tunnels. Serial topography measurements should show reduction in astigmatism and a more regular pattern. The refractive effect of ring implantation stabilises around 3 months post-op.

4.2.4 Combination Procedures

Implantation of intrastromal rings reduces the overall magnitude of corneal astigmatism and makes any remaining astigmatism more regular. If there is significant residual refractive error, this may be corrected with spectacles or contact lenses. Patients who are intolerant of contact lenses may prefer further surgical correction.

Intrastromal ring implantation has been combined with subsequent implantation of a toric phakic intraocular lens which can be custom-made to correct the residual refractive error. It has also been combined with corneal collagen cross-linking in the management of keratoconus. This has the advantage of treating the existing irregular astigmatism as well as addressing the underlying cause and reducing the tendency of the refractive error to progress. Evidence suggests that intrastromal rings should be placed first, followed by cross-linking.

4.3 Refractive Laser Surgery

The introduction of the excimer laser into ophthalmic practice has enabled precision reshaping of the cornea to affect the eye's refractive power and thus correct refractive errors. The excimer (= 'excited dimer') laser operates in the ultraviolet C range, the argon-fluoride laser emitting at 193 nm. This high-energy beam disrupts intermolecular bonds in surface tissues, causing photodisruption without local heating. The result of this photoablative effect is that tissue is 'vaporised' and lost to the atmosphere. Since the energy of the beam is easily absorbed by superficial tissues, it does not penetrate to any depth. With this technology, tissue can be sculpted with sub-micrometre precision.

4.3.1 Patient Selection

The majority of people with focusing errors of the eye are able to have laser vision correction to reduce the need for glasses or contact lenses. Identifying patients who are suitable candidates for refractive surgery and identifying those who are not is a critical skill in successful refractive surgery, and attention should be paid to developing

Table 4.2 Visual outcomes in keratoplasty

Suitable candidates	Unsuitable candidates
Low to moderate myopes (up to −8 D)	*Factors relating to the eye*:
Low to moderate hyperopes (up to +3 D)	Thin corneas for LASIK (thin:<520 µm, unsuitable: <500 µm)
Low to moderate regular astigmatism (<4 D)	Ectasia (especially keratoconus)
Stable refraction (≤0.5 D change in 12 months)	Visually significant cataract
Motivated by spectacle independence but accepting limitations (onset of presbyopia, refractive drift, potential for retreatment etc.)	Unstable refraction
Realistic expectations	Refractive error outside the approved limits
Compliance with aftercare	Abnormally steep cornea ($K>48$ D)
Age 21 years or older	Abnormally flat cornea ($K<40$ D)
Good vision in both eyes with spectacles or contact lenses	Irregular astigmatism
	Corneal pathology, especially scars, previous radial keratotomy, reduced corneal sensation and dystrophies, especially epithelial basement membrane dystrophy
	Poor lid hygiene
	Dry eyes
	Nystagmus
	Amblyopia
	Poor vision in fellow eye
	Very deep set (difficult eye exposure)
	Factors relating to patient's general health:
	Pregnancy or breastfeeding
	Diabetes
	Collagen vascular disease (e.g. SLE, RA)
	Connective tissue disease (e.g. Marfan)
	Factors relating to patient's personality:
	Unreasonable expectations
	Obsessive personality
	Denying or trivialising operational risks
	Unwilling to comply with medication or postoperative follow-up
	Not available for follow-up (patients with challenging schedules)
	Unwillingness to wear reading glasses

this skill early in the refractive surgeon's training. The key areas here are identifying a patient's motivation and expectations, assessing risk factors for postoperative keratectasia and other complications and deciding how to obtain optimal optics.

Key factors can be divided into those relating to the eye, those relating to the patient's systemic health and those relating to the patient's personality (Table 4.2). Also consider co-pathology, especially maculopathies (diabetic, myopic degenerative, etc.) and lens opacifications.

4.3.2 Pre-assessment

The pre-assessment for laser surgery comprises a comprehensive examination always of both eyes and includes a discussion of the patient's visual needs. During the pre-assessment, data necessary for refractive correction is collected. At this time it is also possible to suggest a certain method of correction and to discuss it with the patient, including a risk and benefit assessment. Risks that suggest treatment is inadvisable should also be recognised.

The patient must be encouraged to ask questions and express any concerns before embarking on a course of treatment as it is easier and more constructive to address these at the outset. If the patient wishes to undergo treatment, informed consent must be given and documented, usually on a specific form, and the patient given a copy well in advance of the surgery. The patient should also be given written information about their treatment. Some surgeons will dictate a letter to the patient summarising the consultation, including what was discussed and the benefits and risks of the treatment which is planned.

Refractive stability is usually achieved by age 21 and some surgeons decline to treat patients under this age. The patient's refractive error should have been stable for a year before refractive surgery is carried out. The refractive error at the preoperative visit can be compared to previous spectacle prescriptions to ensure that it has not changed significantly. If a change of more than 0.5 D is seen in 1 year, surgery should be deferred and the patient reassessed at 6-month intervals until stable.

Pre-existing blepharitis and dry eye must be corrected as much as possible before surgery to reduce the risk of intraoperative and postoperative complications (e.g. epithelial abrasion during flap creation and infection/severe dry eye/diffuse lamellar keratitis, respectively).

Patients should be asked to refrain from wearing rigid gas-permeable contact lenses for 3–4 weeks prior to assessment (to aid topography and pachymetry) and from wearing soft contact lenses for 2 weeks.

Assessment of patient's history:

- Motivation and goals
- Occupation
- Leisure/sport activities
- Past ocular history (POH): trauma, infections, inflammations, previous operations
- Past medical history (PMH): diabetes, SLE, RA
- Medications
- Allergies
- Pregnancy/breastfeeding
- Tendency for increased scarring
- Refractive stability
- Use of glasses for distance vision and reading (including varifocals)
- Use of contact lenses: type, frequency
- Dry eyes
- Amblyopia (strabismus, occlusion therapy)

The bilateral examination includes (in the following order):

- Topography (with pachymetry)
- Autorefraction (with keratometry)
- Aberrometry (corneal and ocular wavefront, higher-order aberration)
- Uncorrected distance visual acuity (UDVA)
- Subjective refraction
- Spectacle-corrected distance visual acuity (CDVA)
- Determination of the dominant eye
- Pupillometry: scotopic and photopic
- Topical anaesthesia (G proxymetacaine 0.5 %)
- Tonometry
- Contact pachymetry (ultrasound)
- Dilation (G tropicamide 1 %)
- Slit-lamp examination of the anterior segment: lids, conjunctiva, cornea, lens
- Fundus examination: optic nerve, macula, retinal periphery
- Optional: biometry, corrected and uncorrected near visual acuity, binocular visual acuity, specular microscopy, Schirmer test, cover test, contact lens simulation of monovision

Key points to discuss and for consenting:

- Reasons for surgery (motivation)
- Vision expectations
- Lifestyle, occupation, sports
- Night vision
- Need for glasses and presbyopia (patients in mid-1940s)
- The procedure (anaesthesia, drape, fixation light, noise, smell)
- The first 24 h after the procedure: pain, vision
- Flap complications
- Dry eyes
- Infections
- Visual disturbances: glare, halo, stars
- Aftercare: eye drops, eye protection, do's and don'ts, follow-up regime
- Emergency situations and actions
- Refractive and visual outcomes
- Enhancements

Key points for patients to follow on the day of surgery:

- Contact lenses must not be worn for 2 weeks prior to surgery.
- No eye makeup or perfume (in particular no mascara!) should be used
- Patients are allowed to eat and drink normally
- Patients should take their normal medications

4.3.3 Surgical Planning

Once the pre-assessment has been completed and the patient has decided to proceed with laser vision correction (LASIK or LASEK), the surgeon starts to develop a surgical plan. This is an important step that will require understanding of patients' needs and goals, the use of equipment, the technical limitations and the surgical skills and experience.

Key questions to consider for the surgical plan are:

- What laser mode should be used (wavefront guided, topography guided)?
- What refractive correction should be entered into the excimer laser?
- Is a nomogram adjustment required?
- What is the size of the optical zone?
- What is the accurate flap diameter and thickness?
- For microkeratome use: What suction ring is required?
- What is the thickness of the residual stromal bed?
- What is the predicted postoperative corneal curvature?

The following recommendations should be used as guidance and have to be adjusted to the individually used surgical equipment.

4.3.3.1 What Laser Mode Should Be Used?

The basic treatment profile is a simple spherocylindrical correction. In the past, this treatment profile sometimes was creating a more spherical corneal profile for myopic patients which could induce positive spherical aberration, especially with small optical zones. Most laser ablation profiles now are aspherical and aberration-free and provide great treatment accuracy for patients with regular astigmatism and minimal higher-order aberrations.

Patients with greater amounts of higher-order aberrations may benefit from wavefront-optimised or wavefront-guided treatments.

- Wavefront-optimised (WFO) treatment uses standard adjustments based on population averages to avoid inducing higher-order aberrations during excimer laser refractive surgery. The main objective is to preserve a prolate corneal surface and maintain its asphericity. The visual benefit of this is that the patient may report sharper distance acuity and greater contrast sensitivity. The price paid for this is a slight loss in depth of field (the use of aspheric IOLs in cataract surgery is a direct analogy of this approach). This is suitable for 70–90 % of patients.
- Wavefront-guided (WFG) treatments incorporate a customised adjustment based on the patient's measured wavefront preoperatively. This approach may be most suited to patients with higher than average pre-existing higher-order aberrations. Subtle advantages have been reported with this approach in patients with high pre-op spherical aberration in terms of post-op contrast sensitivity. However, WFG treatments remove more tissue than WFO treatments and are pupil dependent.

When there is significant irregular astigmatism, it may be preferable to base customisation of the ablation profile on the patient's preoperative corneal topography since the irregular astigmatism will be mainly due to abnormalities in the cornea. This is because it is not possible to adequately describe the corneal shape in terms of Zernike polynomials, as is required for wavefront customisations. In such cases, as in instances with large amounts of regular astigmatism, alignment is critical to account for any cyclotorsion on changing from upright to supine. Some laser systems use iris recognition for this, in combination with dynamic eye tracking.

Some excimer operating systems also allow the surgeon to manually customise a proposed ablation after programming for the desired correction and taking into account topography or wavefront data (e.g. z-clip on the Zeiss MEL 80). This gives an extra level of customisation but requires the surgeon to have experience and detailed understanding of the principles involved in order to obtain best results.

Examples

- Most surgeons recommend using wavefront-guided treatments for patients treated with the VI SX S4 excimer laser.
- On the Schwind Amaris platform, wavefront-guided treatments are recommended if the corneal and ocular higher-order aberrations are greater than 0.5 DEq. If the difference between the corneal and ocular higher-order aberration is greater than 0.25 DEq, then an 'ocular wavefront' treatment is recommended; otherwise, a 'corneal wavefront' treatment is used.

4.3.3.2 What Refractive Correction Should Be Entered into the Excimer Laser?

The determination follows the 'principle of minimum risk'. This means, take the measurement with the least negative (most positive) amount of spherical equivalent, take the measurement with the least amount of refractive astigmatism, and if several refractive astigmatisms are equal, take the cylinder measurement closest to with-the-rule.

Further recommendations include: aim for emmetropia for young myopic eyes and consider target of −0.5 D in presbyopes, aim for mild myopia (−0.25 to −0.5) for hyperopic eyes because of the regression tendency, undercorrect cylinder treatments to prevent changes in the cylinder axis, and respect FDA-approved indications and ranges for laser treatments. Generally, it is important to be familiar with the laser system, its performance and with recommended nomogram adjustments.

If the treatment is wavefront guided, choose the wavefront scan that is closest to the subjective refraction. As a rule of thumb, reassess the scans if the difference between the manifest refraction and the wavefront refraction results is more than 0.5 D for the sphere, 0.25 D for the cylinder and 10° for the cylinder axis.

Attempts should be made to identify the patient's dominant eye, and the surgeon may wish to discuss monovision if appropriate. Monovision relies on blur suppression, and not all patients are able to adapt well. A trial of contact lens simulation of monovision is essential before surgical treatment. The nondominant eye is usually corrected for near vision (residual myopia of around −1.75 D is usual) and the dominant eye for distance vision (emmetropia).

4.3.3.3 Is a Nomogram Adjustment Required?

Most laser treatments benefit from nomogram adjustment. This can be done for the spherical equivalent only (e.g. a 5 % boost) or for the sphere and cylinder component separately. Generally, the cylinder axis should not be modified, as wavefront and topography measurements are precise in determining the astigmatic axis. (Comment: subjective refraction does not provide the 'pure cylinder' since it is a combination of cylinder, coma, trefoil and other higher-order aberrations.)

If you start working at a new centre, use the nomogram adjustments that were established by your centre colleagues. Over time, analyse your personal outcomes and modify the nomograms to match your requirements. Always analyse the results carefully when using a new laser or new controller software.

4.3.3.4 What Is the Accurate Flap Diameter and Thickness?

The diameter of a flap depends on the refractive treatment. It must take into account the treatment zone plus the blend zone. For Femtolaser flap creation, a common, universal diameter is 9.5 mm (e.g. Ziemer LDV). With the microkeratome, as a rule of thumb, a diameter of 8.5 mm should be used for all corneas with $K > 45$ mm and a size of 9.5 mm for all other corneas.

Generally, larger flaps are required for hyperopic treatments because of the larger ablation zone. Larger flaps require larger suction rings which might be more difficult to place in smaller and deep set eyes (hyperopes).

For microkeratomes, many surgeons prefer a thickness of the flap between 110 and 140 μm. Thicker flaps may be associated with increased microstriae, while thinner flaps are more difficult to handle for beginners and may be prone to buttonholes.

The thickness of corneal flaps varies between different microkeratomes. Always use new blades when cutting flaps with microkeratomes; sharper blades create thicker flaps. Faster passes (translation velocity) create thinner flaps and thinner corneas create thinner flaps, too. Following cutting the cornea with a microkeratome, surgeons should measure the flap thickness (residual cornea thickness) by ultrasound pachymetry.

The flap creation with a Femtolaser is more flexible and more predictable. Normally, flap thicknesses used for Femto-LASIK are between 90 and 110 μm.

Anterior corneal stroma is different to posterior corneal stroma regarding structural strengths. In the anterior 200–300 μm of the corneal stroma, the collagen fibres cross and interlink more strongly, which provides higher structural integrity to the cornea. Collagen fibres in the posterior 200–300 μm of the stroma are more parallel oriented, resulting in an overall weaker corneal strength. The aim of treatment is to prevent as much uncut anterior stroma as possible. Therefore, corneal flaps should be as thin as possible (thin flaps are more prone to wrinkles and folds).

Examples

- The measured flap thickness was 134 ± 15 μm for the AMO Amadeus microkeratome with an attempted thickness of 140 μm (Solomon, JCRS 2004).
- Flap thickness was 132 ± 23 μm for the Moria M2 with a 110 μm head (Muallem, JCRS 2004).
- The mean standard deviation for Intralase flaps ranged from ±3.2 to ±7.3 μm, depending on the attempted flap thickness, which was set between 90 and 110 μm (Prakash, JRS 2010).

4.3.3.5 What Suction Ring Is Required (Microkeratome)?

The size of the suction ring and stop position is determined by the steepest keratometry reading and the desired flap diameter. The correct sizes can be obtained from tables and nomograms provided by the microkeratome manufacturer.

Example

- To create a 9.5 mm diameter flap with the Moria M2 in a cornea with 42 D steepest *K*, the ring size is '−1' and the stop position is '8.0'. Always check the labelling carefully before starting the flap creation.

4.3.3.6 What Is the Size of the Optical Zone?

The optical (and transition) zone is mainly determined by the preoperative refractive error (myopia or hyperopia) and the size of the scotopic pupil.

A standard optical zone for the treatment of myopic eyes is between 6 and 6.5 mm. Hyperopic and astigmatic eyes require larger overall treatment zones that can range up to 7 mm, depending on the transition zone (overall optical zones can be 9.5 mm in diameter).

Generally, the area of ablation should be greater than the scotopic pupil size to avoid optical aberrations such as haloes and poor night vision, which arise when light refracted at the edge of the treatment zone enters the pupil. A blend or transition zone is used at the edge of the optical zone rather than having a sudden transition between treated and untreated cornea. The size of the LASIK flap must therefore take into account the optical zone plus the transition zone.

On the other hand, the larger the chosen optical zone, the more tissue must be removed to achieve a given correction. This is particularly important when planning a large correction or in eyes with thinner corneas.

Examples

- On the VISX S4 platform, typical optical/transition zones are 6/8 mm for myopia with a pupil size <6 mm scotopic, 6.5/8.5 mm for myopia with a pupil size of 6 mm or more, and 6/9 mm for hyperopia.
- On the Schwind Amaris platform, typical optical zones are 6.3 mm for myopia, 6.7 mm for hyperopia and 7 mm for astigmatism.

4.3.3.7 What Is the Thickness of the Residual Stromal Bed?

The thickness of untreated stroma remaining at the bed of the cornea after ablation (=residual stromal bed, RSB) must remain above a critical value in order for the cornea to retain its structural integrity and reduce the risk of posttreatment ectasia. Over the years, the recommendations for minimal RSB have increased from 200 to 250 μm (still common) and now 300 μm (used by most surgeons).

The excimer laser's computer will calculate the thickness of tissue to be removed for the programmed treatment, and the surgeon must check that sufficient corneal stroma remains. If the RSB is lower than 300 μm, a surface-based treatment or an alternative to excimer laser should be considered. The RSB can be estimated preoperatively:

$$\text{RSB} = \text{Central corneal thickness}\left(\text{CCT}\right)\ \text{pre-op} - \text{Flap thickness} - \text{Ablation depth}$$

Examples

- A myopic patient with 550 μm CCT needs 4 D of spherical equivalent (SE) correction. A Femtolaser is used for the flap creation (110 μm). On the VISX platform, each SE dioptre of myopic treatment equals 12 μm (with 6 mm optical zone) or 15 μm (with 6.5 mm optical zone) or 18 μm (with 6.5 mm optical zone with wavefront); an additional 8 μm have to be added for an 8 mm transition zone. In this example, with a 6/8 mm optical/transition zone, the estimated RSB is $550-110-(4\times12+8)=384$ μm.
- The same patient as above is treated with the Schwind Amaris laser. For an optical zone of 6.3 mm (myopic treatment), an average of 15.4 μm per SE dioptre is used to calculate the ablation depth. This increases to 17.4 μm/D in hyperopes (6.7 mm optical zone) and 20.9 μm/D in astigmatic patients (7 mm optical zone). The estimated RSB is $550-110-(4\times15.4)=378.4$ μm.

4.3.3.8 What Is the Predicted Postoperative Corneal Curvature?

To estimate the postoperative corneal curvature for highly myopic patients, multiply the preoperative spherical equivalent by 0.75 and subtract this product from the average of the preoperative keratometric value. Although controversial, it is wise to keep the postoperative corneal curvature above 35 D.

Example

The estimated postoperative K of a patient with a preoperative refraction of $-6.25+0.5\times90°$ (SE = −6 D) and a preoperative average K of 41 D is $41-(6\times0.75)=36.5$ D.

4.3.4 Technique of LASIK

Laser-assisted in situ keratomileusis (LASIK, Fig. 4.3) enables the surgeon to modify the refractive power of the cornea by laser ablation of corneal stroma (Fig. 4.4) after creation of a hinged flap. There are a number of differences between this true flap-based refractive procedure and the surface-based procedures described below in terms of patient selection, risks and benefits of the procedure and post-op recovery. A flap is created using a microkeratome or a femtosecond laser.

4.3.4.1 Preparation

The patient is positioned beneath the excimer laser, and eyelash drapes and a speculum are applied under topical anaesthesia. The cornea is dried and ink marks applied to guide accurate flap alignment at the end of the procedure.

4.3.4.2 Flap Creation

- If a microkeratome is used for the flap creation, this is done under the microscope of the excimer laser. The suction ring is applied, taking care to centre it at the desired location and that adequate fixation has been achieved. The suction generates such a high IOP that the central retinal artery is temporarily occluded and the iris becomes ischaemic. The patient's vision dims and the pupil dilates slightly. The IOP may be checked with a Barraquer tonometer. The microkeratome is advanced to create the flap and reversed. The suction is released and the suction ring/microkeratome assembly is removed from the eye. The patient's vision returns.

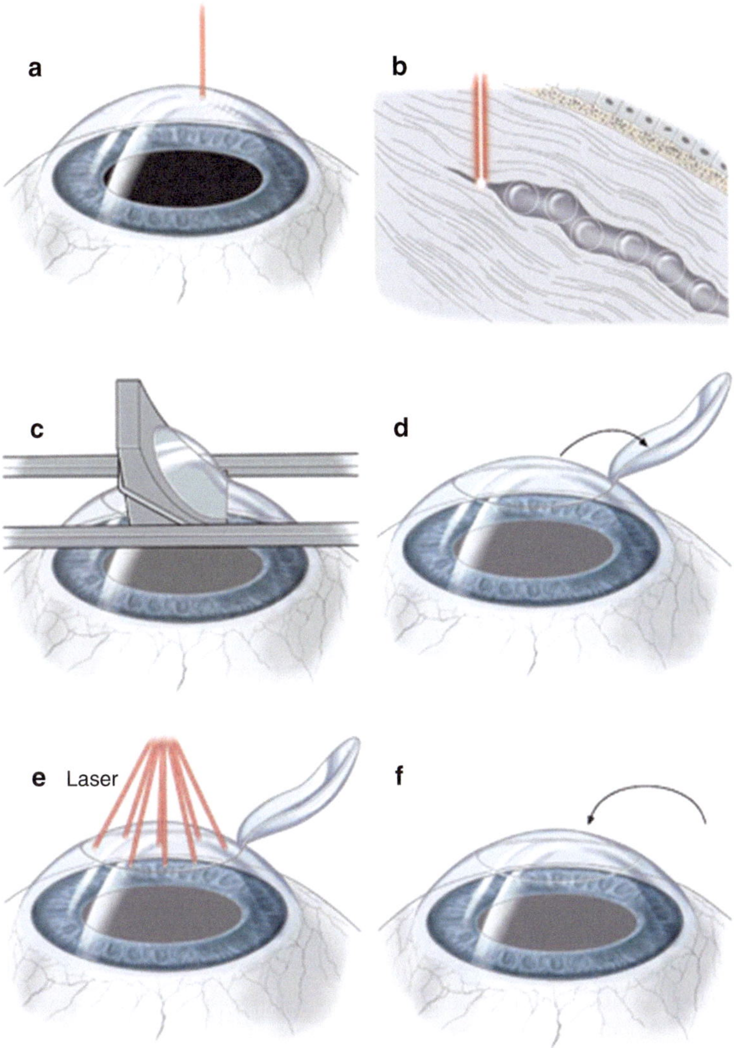

Fig. 4.3 Illustration of the technique of LASIK. (**a**, **b**) femtosecond laser flap creation; (**c**) microkeratome flap creation; (**d**) reflection of flap; (**e**) application of excimer laser to stromal bed; (**f**) replacement of flap

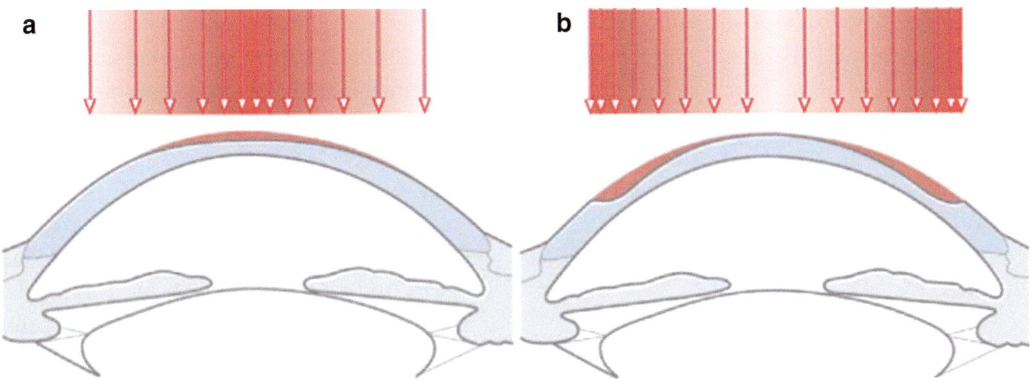

Fig. 4.4 Illustration of excimer laser ablation profiles for myopia (**a**) and hyperopia (**b**)

- If a femtosecond laser is used, this usually requires flap creation with the Femtolaser and subsequent transfer of the patient to the excimer laser. This procedure is sometimes called IntraLASIK or Femto-LASIK. The individual steps are similar to the microkeratome use, starting with the placement of a suction ring. Using the AMO Intralase FS60 or iFS Femtolaser, this ring is placed on the eye, and the laser head is then 'docked' to the ring for flap creation. The suction ring is integrated in the hand-held laser delivery unit of the LDV Femtolaser, which is applied to the eye before flap creation. This manoeuvrable system allows patients to be treated on the patient bed of the excimer laser and without having to be relocated.

4.3.4.3 Laser Ablation

The flap is assessed for quality and centration, and if the surgeon is satisfied with both, it is lifted with a spatula to expose the stromal bed. The bed can be dried with spears to ensure an optimal surface for ablation and a small piece of sponge used to protect the hinge for accidental ablation. The eye tracker is activated and the laser ablation profile is applied.

4.3.4.4 Finalising

The stromal bed is gently irrigated with chilled BSS and the flap is replaced carefully, ensuring it is aligned with the marks placed at the outset. At this stage it is essential to avoid both over-hydrating the tissues and exerting tension on the flap which would create microstriae. Excess fluid is removed from the interface by absorbent spears at the flap edge, and preservative-free antibiotic and steroid eye drops are given. A bandage contact lens is not required if there have been no intraoperative difficulties with the flap. The eye is protected with a clear shield. The flap should be checked at the slit lamp before the patient is discharged to ensure it has remained in the correct place, and postoperative eye drops are given according to the surgeon's preference.

4.3.4.5 Aftercare

Typically, this would include (preservative-free) antibiotic, tear supplements and steroid. Topical NSAID and oral analgesia may also be given. The patient may be advised to rest with their eyes closed as much as possible for the remainder of the day since the topical anaesthesia used for the surgery will reduce the blink rate, leading to dry eyes and greater discomfort.

4.3.4.6 Review

The patient should be reviewed the next day for any early signs of diffuse lamellar keratitis and to check the flap position. Some surgeons review the patient at 48–72 h for signs of infection or dry eye. Subsequent follow-up is dictated by the surgeon's preference and any postoperative difficulties which may occur but should include a subjective refraction at 1–2 months. Collection of postoperative refractive outcomes, including topography (Fig. 4.5), is vital for clinical audit and to refine the treatment nomograms for greater surgical accuracy.

4.3.5 Surface Treatments (PRK and LASEK)

Photorefractive keratectomy (PRK) was the first form of excimer laser refractive surgery introduced clinically (around 1989 by Marshall and Gartry in the UK). Variations of the technique (LASEK, EPI-LASIK, Trans-PRK) are now included under the term 'surface treatments' as there is little difference between them.

4.3.5.1 Preparation

Laser refractive surgery is performed under topical anaesthesia as the patient's cooperation is required for them to fixate on the target light so that the refractive treatment can be applied accurately. Adhesive drapes exclude the lashes from the operative field to reduce the risk of infection, and a speculum is used to hold the eye open.

4.3.5.2 Epithelial Removal

- In PRK the epithelium is removed over the area to be treated by rubbing with sponge spears and a hockey-stick blade. If available, the laser's slit-lamp accessory may be useful to identify small residual islands of epithelium which must be removed.
- In Trans-PRK the epithelium is removed by the excimer laser (trans-epithelial, 50 μm) instead of manual debridement. This can be

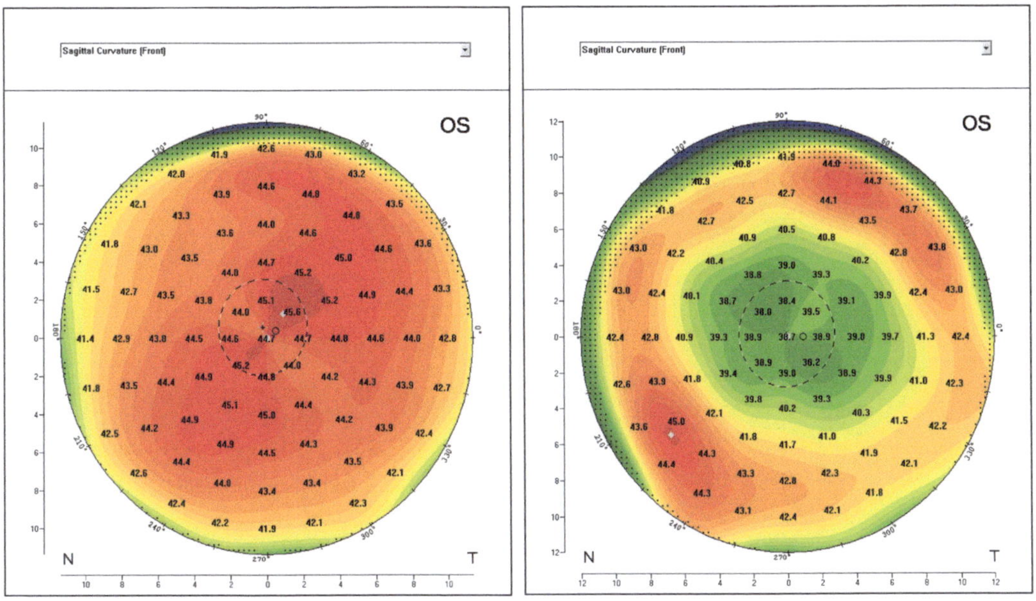

Fig. 4.5 Change in corneal topography (Pentacam) in myopic LASIK for (7 D)

useful if the ablation profile is topography guided as the surface profile to which the treatment is customised is effectively transferred to the exposed stroma.

- In LASEK (laser-assisted epithelial keratomileusis), the epithelium is removed or folded as a sheet (epithelial layer) following application of 20 % alcohol for 30 s with a well (Fig. 4.6). After the stromal ablation, this sheet is then replaced to its original position. The proposed benefit of this is the modification of the healing response and the reduction of stromal reaction to cytokines. However, the technique by which the epithelium is removed effectively devitalises the epithelium so many surgeons feel that replacing this has no benefit.
- Epi-LASEK is a modified LASEK procedure where a superficial layer of epithelium is separated by an epi-microkeratome (Moria or Zyoptix XP). This can be done with or without previous application of alcohol to the epithelium. The peeled epithelium then can be replaced on the stroma after ablation.

4.3.5.3 Laser Ablation

The exposed stroma is dried and the eye tracker activated. The programmed ablation profile is then applied.

4.3.5.4 Mitomycin C

Mild stromal haze is sometimes seen after surface laser treatment, indicating activation of keratocytes in the healing process. This is particularly noticeable after treatment of larger refractive errors and may limit the subsequent BCVA so moderation of this may be desirable. This is achieved by using mitomycin C (0.2 mg/ml) applied after the laser ablation for 15–60 s to reduce keratocyte activation and subsequent fibroblast activity and scarring. The mitomycin is wiped onto the central cornea using a spear, taking care to avoid it running off and coming into contact with the limbal cells. After 30 s it is wiped off with dry spears and the surface of the eye is irrigated thoroughly with cold BSS. The used spears and irrigation fluid must be contained within a suitable drape and disposed of as hazardous material by incineration.

4.3.5.5 Finalising

Topical (preservative-free) antibiotic and steroid eye drops are given and a bandage contact lens is placed; the speculum and drapes are removed.

4.3.5.6 Aftercare

Postoperatively, the patient is instructed not to rub the eye and to instil drops of antibiotic, steroid and lubricant according to the surgeon's preference.

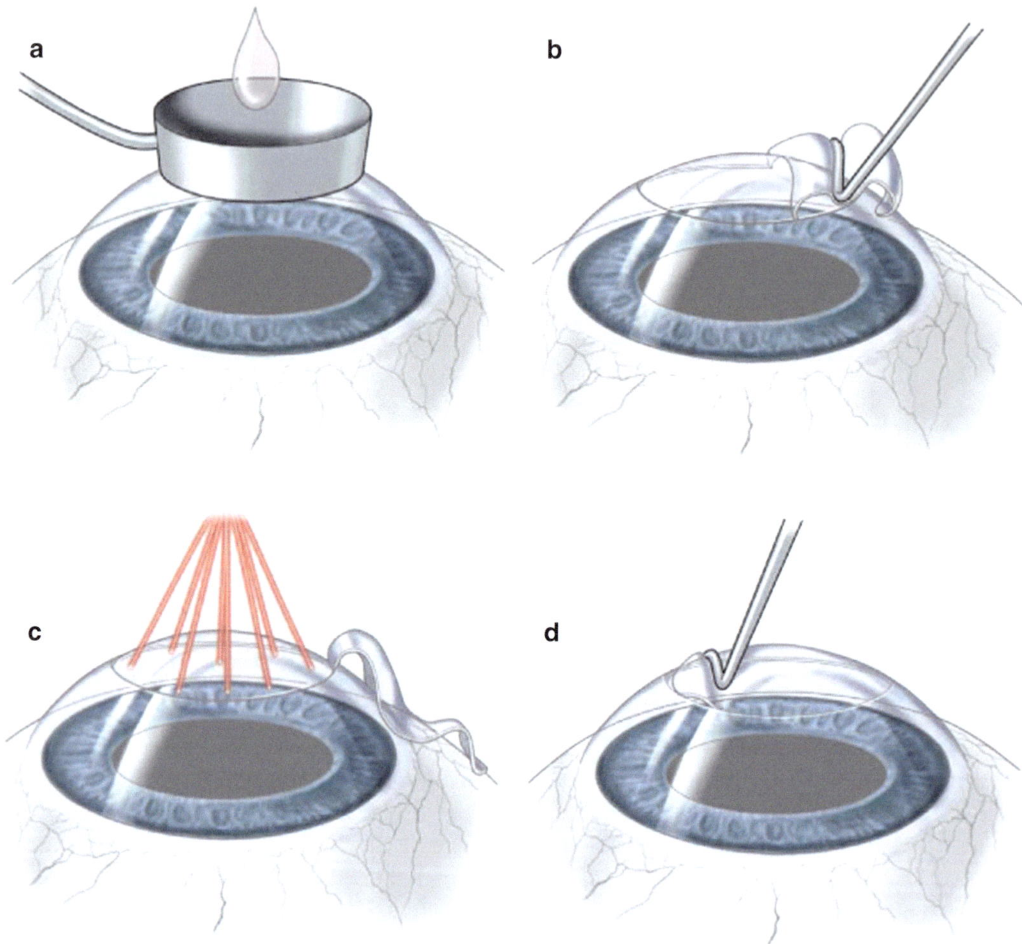

Fig. 4.6 Illustration of LASEK. (**a**) application of ethanol to cornea in well; (**b**) reflection of epithelial flap; (**c**) application of excimer laser to stromal surface; (**d**) replacement of epithelium

A topical NSAID and oral analgesia can also be prescribed. The fellow eye may be treated on the same day or on another occasion. The patient may be advised to rest with their eyes closed as much as possible for the remainder of the day since the topical anaesthesia used for the surgery will reduce the blink rate, leading to dry eyes and greater discomfort.

4.3.5.7 Review

The patient should be reviewed the next day and again within 5–7 days to check for signs of infection (very rare), monitor recovery and ensure compliance with the topical medication. Vision is often slow to recover with surface ablations and the patient must be warned about this during the preoperative consultation. The bandage contact lens is removed at day 5–7 and the epithelium assessed. If adequate healing has occurred, it may be left out; if it is slow to heal or the patient has significant dry eye or discomfort, it may be replaced and reassessed a week later. A subjective refraction can be performed around a month after surgery, although stabilisation may take several months.

4.3.6 Aftercare

After the laser procedure, a significant improvement in vision is often experienced within hours and much improved following sleep. Patients are

Table 4.3 Standard drug regime for Femto-LASIK

Medication	Frequency and duration
G levofloxacin 0.5 % (Oftaquix®)	qds for 1–2 weeks
G dexamethasone 0.1 % (Maxidex®)	hourly for 2 days 2 hourly for 1 week qds for 2 weeks bd for 1 week
G sodium hyaluronate 0.15 % (Oxyal®)	2 hourly for 2 days qds for 1 months then PRN
Pain relief (optional)	PO paracetamol max. 4 g/day G proxymetacaine 0.5 % (Minims)

Table 4.4 Standard drug regime for LASEK/PRK

Medication	Frequency and duration
G levofloxacin 0.5 % (Oftaquix®)	tds until removal of CL (+1 day)
G dexamethasone 0.1 % (Maxidex®)	tds for 4 weeks
G sodium hyaluronate 0.15 % (Oxyal®)	2 hourly for 2 days tds for 1 months then PRN
G ketorolac 0.5 % (Acular®)	tds until removal of CL (+1 day)
PO mefenamic acid 250 mg (Ponstan®)	tds for 5 days
Contact lens (CL)	e.g. PureVision, 8.6 mm, for 1 week
Pain relief (optional)	PO paracetamol max. 4 g/day G proxymetacaine 0.5 % (Minims)

usually able to return to work after 48 h. Vision improves more rapidly after Femto-LASIK than with LASEK treatments. A common standard regime for Femto-LASIK and LASEK/PRK is shown in Tables 4.3 and 4.4.

Information for the patient for the time after LASIK/LASEK:

- Keep your eyes closed in as relaxed a manner as possible for 2 h (as if you were asleep). Blink frequently for the rest of the time.
- Do not squeeze your eyes and do not rub your eyes for 1 week.
- It is essential that you wear the protective shield for the first week.
- On the first day, you can have a shower, but wash your face carefully.
- After 1 week you may wear make-up again.
- Sport: No individual sports for 1 week. No team sports or ball sports for 2 weeks. No contact sports for 4 weeks. No diving for 2 weeks.
- UV radiation: No holidays by the sea or in the mountains for 2 weeks. No solarium for 4 weeks. Wear sunglasses with good UV protection in the case of strong solar radiation.
- Visiting public swimming pools and saunas is not recommended for 2 weeks.
- In the first few days, avoid rooms where people are smoking or cleaning.
- Apply the eye drops in the prescribed dosage to improve the surgical result.
- Inform your surgeon of any medication intolerances you may have.
- If you have any complaints, please inform the surgeon immediately! Notify the doctor in particular if any of the following occur: pain, acute loss of vision or increased redness of the eyes.

4.3.7 Intraoperative Complications

With meticulous technique, the risk of complications during refractive surgery can be minimised but not eliminated. The increased complexity of LASIK over LASEK also increases the risks of complications, which are mainly related to the corneal flap and its creation. An overview of intra- and postoperative complications of LASIK and LASEK is shown in the Table 4.5.

4.3.7.1 Incomplete Flap

Incomplete flaps are due to a premature termination of the microkeratome, for example, following obstruction by lids/lashes or loss of suction. The microkeratome should be reversed and removed from the eye. The flap must be left to heal. The patient can be offered surface laser treatment at a later date.

4.3.7.2 Thin Flap

If inadequate suction is achieved, a thin flap may result, which is harder to manipulate safely and more prone to wrinkles. It may be possible to

Table 4.5 Summary of intra- and postoperative complications

Intraoperative complications	Postoperative complications
LASIK:	LASIK and LASEK:
Incomplete flap	Dry eyes (LASIK>LASEK)
Thin flap	Infectious keratitis
Buttonhole flap	Ectasia (LASIK>LASEK)
Full-thickness flap	Corneal haze (LASEK>LASIK)
Free cap	Night vision problems
Decentred flap	Glare, halos, stars
Limbal bleeding	Significant under- and overcorrection
Interface debris	Loss of best-corrected vision
Epithelial defects	
Poorly adhering flap	LASIK:
	Epithelial Ingrowth
Femto-LASIK	Flap melt
Opaque bubble layer (OBL)	Flap displacement
Gas breakthrough	Microstriae
	Macrostriae
	Diffuse lamellar keratitis (DLK)
	Transient light sensitivity (TLS)
	In relation to expectations:
	Need for (distance) glasses

complete the treatment under a thin flap as long as there is no buttonhole, but great care must be taken when replacing it.

4.3.7.3 Buttonholed Flap

This describes the case when the microkeratome blade starts a flap but then proceeds up though the epithelium to the surface and then down again towards its intended trajectory. It is more likely to happen in steep corneas. Ablation must not be carried out on the residual epithelial island. The flap must be replaced and allowed to heal. Again, surface laser at a later date may be offered.

4.3.7.4 Full-Thickness Flap

This is the opposite of a buttonholed flap, in that the microkeratome blade enters the anterior chamber during flap creation. This is a risk with older-style microkeratomes if the plate is not properly positioned; newer models have fixed plates which should prevent this. Flaps created with the femtosecond laser are very unlikely to cause this complication if programmed correctly.

4.3.7.5 Free Cap

If the microkeratome cleaves the flap completely from the cornea, it fails to leave a hinge and a free cap results. The risk for a free cap is increased in flat corneas and when suction is inadequate. Stromal ablation may be performed if the exposed stroma is well centred and of a suitable size. The free cap must be replaced with accurate alignment (use of the marks placed at the beginning) to prevent inducing large amounts of irregular astigmatism and enough drying time allowed after repositioning for it to adhere firmly. A bandage contact lens should be used.

4.3.7.6 Decentred Flap

Decentration of the flap may happen when the suction ring slips slightly as suction is being applied to the eye. Ablation to the hinge and the backside of the flap should be avoided to prevent doubly treated areas.

4.3.7.7 Limbal Bleeding

Limbal bleeding is not uncommon and happens more often if the flap is decentred. After adequate wait (30–60 s) and cleaning of the stromal bed, the laser ablation can be performed.

4.3.7.8 Interface Debris

Debris may be trapped under the flap even after thorough irrigation during surgery. The risk is higher if there is pre-existing meibomian gland dysfunction so every effort should be made to correct this preoperatively. Fortunately, this is usually not visually significant.

4.3.7.9 Epithelial Defects

These can occur during the microkeratome pass if the surface of the cornea is not sufficiently lubricated. Preservative-free antibiotic or anaesthetic should be used for this and not BSS as the latter could eventually cause precipitates on the gears and jam the microkeratome. This does not usually have a significant adverse effect on outcome, but a bandage contact lens is recommended for comfort at the end of the procedure, and closer follow-up is needed to observe for signs of flap oedema, DLK and flap melt.

4.3.7.10 Poorly Adhering Flap

This happens if the corneal flap is over-hydrated following excessive irrigation of the flap interface. Sometimes the flap is displaced due to a trauma from the removal of the speculum. Consider replacing the flap in theatre and inserting a bandage contact lens. Insist that the patient wears a shield or glasses after the surgery.

4.3.7.11 Opaque Bubble Layer (OBL)

This complication is unique to femtosecond lasers. Clinically, white areas with fluffy white borders develop during the flap creation. OBL can make pupil visualisation difficult and disable eye tracking. Mild OBL can be 'wiped away', while denser OBL will absorb within 30min, allowing the procedure to be performed after resolution. However, OBL seems not to change the refractive predictability and final outcome.

4.3.7.12 Gas Breakthrough

During the Femtolaser flap creation, small gas bubbles can break through the anterior stroma and be deposited under the epithelium or Bowman's layer. This complication is more common in thin flaps (e.g. 90 μm) and larger diameter flaps in patients with relatively small corneas. If the sub-epithelial bubble is large, the lamellar plane is incomplete underneath the bubble and the corneal flap cannot be lifted. At this stage the procedure should be abandoned. It can be repeated 1–2 months later, cutting a thicker flap or converting to a surface treatment.

4.3.8 Postoperative Complications

Many of the more severe postoperative complications, such as infectious keratitis or dry eyes, can affect the operated eye independent of the procedure. LASIK patients are at risk of flap and interface complications, while LASEK patients have a higher risk of corneal haze (Fig. 4.7) and loss of best-corrected visual acuity.

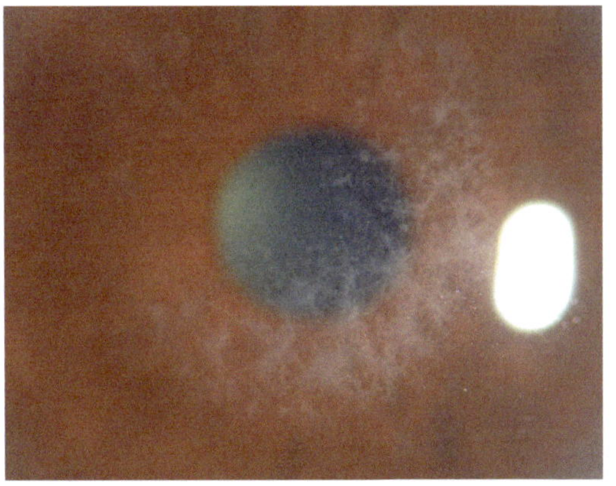

Fig. 4.7 Central corneal scar 6 months after LASEK

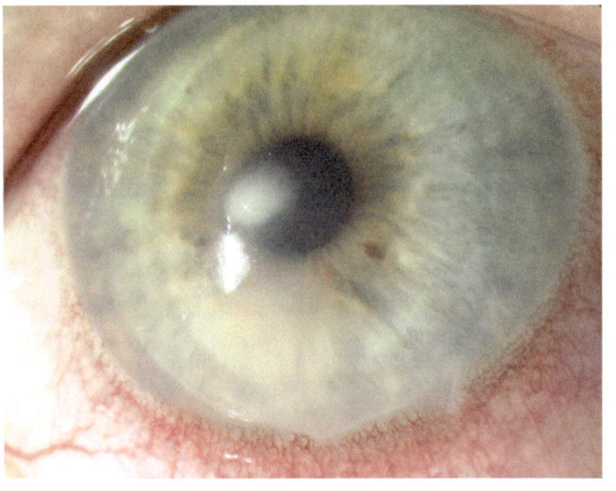

Fig. 4.8 Infectious keratitis after LASIK

4.3.8.1 Dry Eyes

The most common complication of laser vision correction is dry eyes due to the damage to the corneal nerves. This is more likely after LASIK so patients with mild dry eye preoperatively, surface laser may be preferred. Most patients will experience some degree of dry eye after laser refractive surgery, but this usually resolves after 6–12 months as the corneal nerves regenerate. During this time, the patient must use regular tear supplements to prevent discomfort, infection and flap melting. Punctal plugs should be considered. Occasionally, the dryness persists and can have a significant negative effect on quality of life.

4.3.8.2 Infectious Keratitis

This is a severe complication but fortunately rare, reported in about 1:3,000 LASIK procedures (Figs. 4.8 and 4.9). The organisms responsible

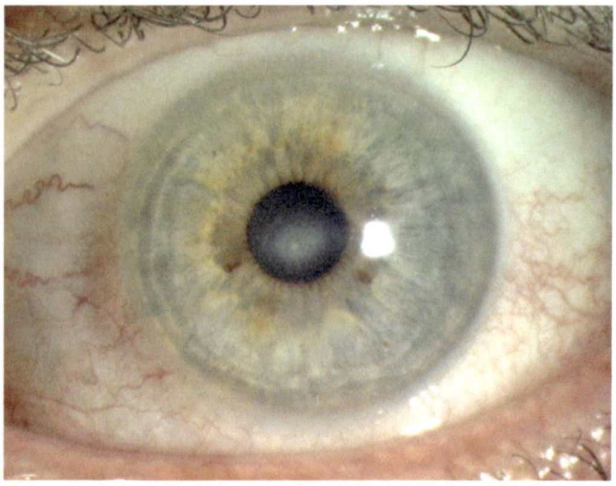

Fig. 4.9 Six weeks of treatment for infectious keratitis after LASIK (same patients as Fig. 4.8)

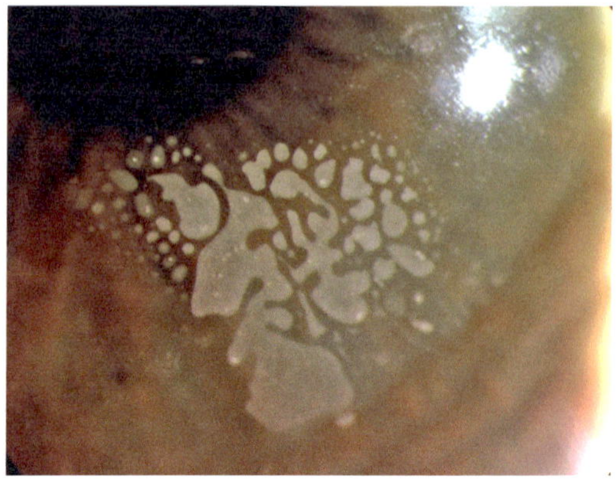

Fig. 4.10 Epithelial ingrowth after LASIK

have been reported as *Mycobacterium*, fungi, *Staphylococcus aureus*, *Streptococcus viridans*, *Streptococcus pneumoniae* and coagulase-negative staphylococci. Symptoms include pain, redness, watering and reduced vision. Examination findings include haze in the interface (but also affecting the stroma), infiltrate with ring of oedema, anterior chamber reaction (cells, hypopyon), sometimes epithelial or flap defects, and hyperaemia. Gram-positive infections, often single infiltrates with distinct margins, are typically seen at the edge of the flap and present in the early postoperative period (3–5 days postoperatively). Those due to Mycobacteria and fungi present after 2–4 weeks with single or multiple lesions in the flap interface, often with indistinct margins. Cultures should be taken and inoculated onto a wide range of media. The flap should be lifted and irrigated. Generally, the complication should be treated like a corneal ulcer. Many surgeons start the treatment with a combination of G levofloxacin (or moxifloxacin 1 %) hourly day and night for 24 h, and then 6×/day, and G amikacin 1.4 % hourly day and night for 24 h, and then 2 hourly. Specific aggressive topical antimicrobial therapy must be directed according to pathogens and sensitivities identified. Daily follow-up is essential.

4.3.8.3 Diffuse Lamellar Keratitis (DLK)

Diffuse lamellar keratitis, also known as diffuse interface keratitis, is a non-specific inflammatory reaction to provoking antigens at the interface. It usually presents on the first or second postoperative day with normal or slightly reduced vision and a faint granular appearance at the interface. DLK is graded according to its clinical appearance (Table 4.6). The inflammation is progressive so early intervention is necessary. If signs are mild (grades 1–2), increasing topical steroids is sufficient. For more advanced forms (3–4), the flap should be lifted and the interface irrigated with BSS. Intensive topical steroid is also required. If existent, also treat blepharitis, epithelial defects and infectious keratitis.

4.3.8.4 Flap Melt

Inflammation due to epithelial abrasion, dry eye, infection or DLK can all lead to release of collagenases which cause melting of the flap. The cause should be identified early and treated aggressively.

4.3.8.5 Dislocated Flap

This can be early or late. Early dislocation may be due to rubbing the eye before the flap has healed sufficiently. The flap should be lifted and repositioned, taking care to clear any epithelium from the flap and stromal bed which might lead to epithelial ingrowth. Late dislocation requires significant force and usually only follows moderate to significant trauma as the interface has usually healed firmly. The risk of striae is significant and early repositioning is mandatory.

Table 4.6 Diffuse lamellar keratitis

Grade	Signs and symptoms	Incidence	Treatment
1.	White granular cells (infiltrate) in the flap periphery, sparing the visual axis, early onset (day 1)	2–4 %	G prednisolone 1 % hourly Follow-up within 1–2 days
2.	Migration of white granular cells into the visual axis (day 2–3). Sometimes decreased visual acuity	0.5 %	G prednisolone 1 % hourly Follow-up next day
3.	Aggregation of dense clumps of white cells in the centre of the visual axis	0.2 %	G prednisolone 1 % hourly
	Reduced visual acuity. Increased risk of scarring		PO prednisolone 60 mg/D Flap lift and brush of stromal bed Culture Follow-up next day
4.	Severe keratitis with dense, central, white infiltrates with (or without) melting. Causes permanent scarring, visual loss and hyperopic shift	1:5,000	Same as grade 3

4.3.8.6 Epithelial Ingrowth

Epithelial cells which gain access to the flap interface can proliferate and migrate centripetally (Fig. 4.10). Ingrowth may occur after primary LASIK, flap lift re-treatment, buttonhole flap complication or trauma. Risk factors include: male, hyperopic preoperative refraction and age >40 years. The visual axis is only rarely affected, but this may cause irregular astigmatism and reduction in acuity. Rarely, epithelial cells may interfere with nutritional supply to the overlying flap and cause melting. If this occurs, the flap should be lifted and the epithelial cells removed by scraping.

4.3.8.7 Ectasia

Ectasia describes the progressive myopia and irregular astigmatism which results from a loss of structural integrity in the cornea after LASIK. This has been diagnosed as early as 1 week post-LASIK as well as after several years (average 12–18 months) and manifests as changing refractive error and poor vision which is difficult to correct with spectacles (Fig. 4.11). It is fortunately rare and can be minimised by strict adherence to recommended patient selection process; however, it can occur spontaneously. Once identified there are a number of treatment options aimed at halting progression and correcting refractive errors. A combination of cross-linking and surface excimer laser has been shown to give good results. If this fails a corneal transplant may be necessary (DALK or PKP).

4.3.8.8 Transient Light Sensitivity Syndrome (TLSS)

TLSS is linked with higher amounts of energy used for the Femtolaser flap creation (less common with the latest lasers), causing photosensitivity at day and night, starting about 1 month after LASIK. Slit-lamp examination is unremarkable and best-corrected visual acuity is usually not affected. Treatment is with topical steroid qds for 1 month.

4.3.9 Enhancements

A minority of patients undergoing refractive surgery will not achieve complete correction of their refractive error with the initial surgery. The risk for this has been estimated at 1 % per dioptre of correction for myopia and slightly higher for corrections of hyperopia. Once the refraction is observed to be stable (usually at 3–6 months), further surgery to correct the residual refractive error can be offered. A rule of thumb is to wait 1 month for each dioptre of initial refractive error/treatment.

Retreatment can be in the form of surface treatment or, for previous LASIK treatment, a flap lift retreatment. Once again, the surgeon

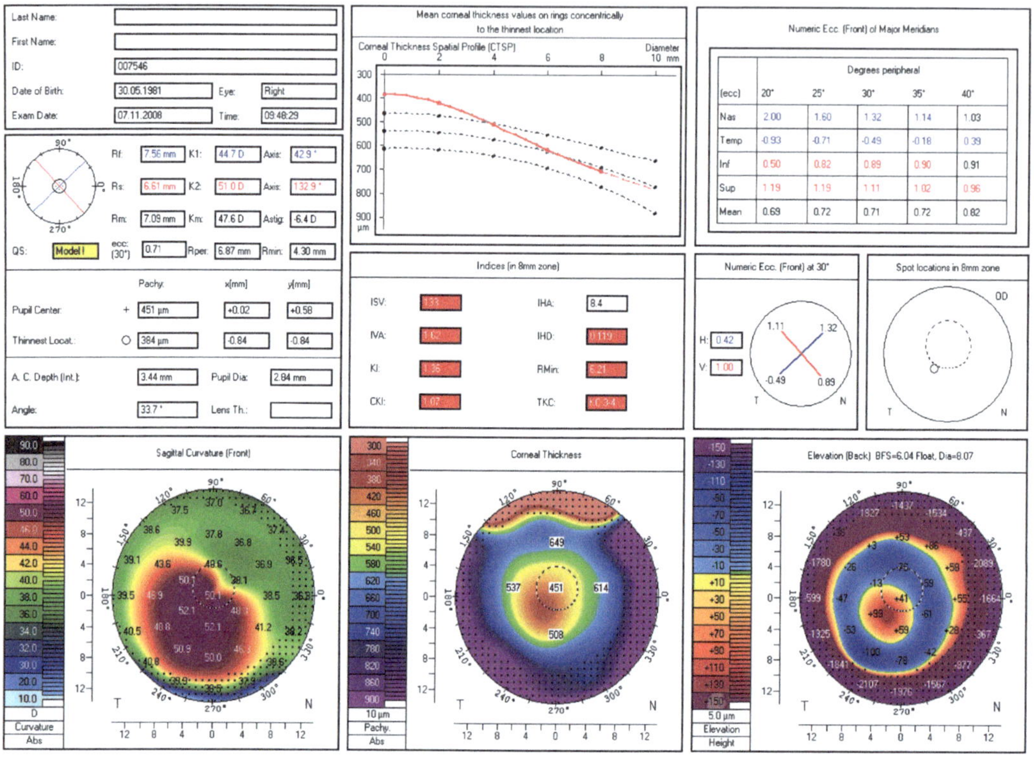

Fig. 4.11 Ectasia (Pentacam)

must ensure that there will be at least 250 μm (better 300 μm) of residual stromal bed. If there is insufficient stroma for treating the bed of the previous LASIK flap, a surface treatment will be necessary.

A LASIK flap can be lifted up to around 10 years or more after the initial treatment; after about 2 years, it will have attached firmly to the bed and attempts to lift it may cause damage. To lift a flap it is best marked at the slit lamp as the optics of the excimer unit's microscope are usually not good enough to visualise the flap edge. The white ring which is visible at the edge of a healed LASIK flap is actually just inside the flap edge so the surgeon must locate the flap edge just outside the white ring. Once it has been marked adequately, the patient is prepared as before for the excimer laser. A 23G needle can be used to lift the epithelium at the flap edge and free the flap around a short arc away from the hinge. Once a free edge is elevated, it can be grasped with fine forceps and the flap lifted with a sweeping movement. If the epithelium at the edge is ragged, it should be gently pushed away from the interface to reduce the risk of subsequent ingrowth. The treatment protocol is applied as before and the flap replaced. The postoperative medication and follow-up regime are as for primary LASIK.

Retreatment by cutting a new flap has been described, but this carries the risks of free, perforated or thin flaps and of creating loose wedges of stromal tissue. It is therefore no longer widely favoured.

Surface ablation for retreatment avoids the risks involved in flap lifting but is associated with the risks of primary surface ablation, namely, discomfort, slower visual recovery and haze. The surgeon must decide in conjunction with the patient which procedure is most appropriate.

Every re-treatment bears the risk of additional loss of best-corrected visual acuity, epithelial ingrowth, striae and other complications.

4.4 Equipment for Corneal Flap Creation

4.4.1 Microkeratomes

Mechanical microkeratomes have a long pedigree and have been constantly refined to improve their accuracy and safety. A suction ring is applied to the surface of the eye and the microkeratome head unit is mounted on the suction ring. The surgeon must select both an appropriate size suction ring and the depth at which the blade cuts the flap. For a steep cornea ($K>45$ D), a smaller ring is used.

Precise gears drive the applanation head across the cornea, flattening it so that the oscillating blade mounted within the unit can cut a flap. The ideal flap is of the desired thickness, of uniform profile and free from abrasions, buttonholes and free caps. Very high intraocular pressures (>60 mmHg) may be generated during these steps. The head motor is reversed to back the blade out from under the flap, and the suction unit/microkeratome assembly is removed from the globe. The flap is then lifted and the exposed stromal bed is ablated. The microkeratome motor is set so that a hinged flap is created; excessive travel in early models resulted in free caps which had to be replaced accurately to avoid inducing irregular astigmatism. Extremes of corneal curvature also risk complications in flap creation: steep corneas with $K>48$ D are at increased risk of buttonholed flaps, and flat corneas ($K<40$ D) are at increased risk of a free cap.

Care must be taken to apply the suction ring precisely so that the resultant flap is centred on the desired spot; if this is misaligned, the ablation profile still can be centred, but there is a risk of the overall ablation diameter being beyond the edge of the bed, resulting in halos and ghosting. If the surgeon is not happy with the location or quality of the flap, it is important to abort the procedure, allow time for the flap to heal and reschedule the patient for an alternative procedure, usually a surface laser treatment after stabilisation (3–6 months).

Care must also be taken to ensure that the suction ring is not applied over conjunctiva. This could lead to pseudosuction, chemosis and unstable fixation of the microkeratome. There is then a high risk of suction break or blade movement during flap creation.

A range of mechanical microkeratomes are available, each with their own characteristics. The way in which the blade is propelled across the cornea varies slightly between models. Some are driven along a straight track forwards and backwards (Amadeus, NIDEK MK-2000, Moria One Use-Plus), some rotate about a pivot (Hansatome, Moria M2) and some act as a pendulum and describe a slightly concave trajectory, applanating the central cornea more than the periphery (e.g. Carriazo-Pendular, Schwind).

4.4.1.1 Bausch & Lomb Hansatome and Zyoptix XP

The Hansatome pivots around a post to create a superior hinged flap. Flaps tend to be slightly thinner than the blade rating, especially for thin corneas. An adapter is used to set up the assembly for right or left eyes.

The successor to the Hansatome, the Zyoptix XP, offers a number of improvements, particularly in the low variability in flap thickness. The orientation of the head assembly can be changed from right eye to left eye simply by moving a switch rather than having to reassemble the unit. The Zyoptix XP is also felt to offer more reliable suction, better centration and smoother flap beds than the Hansatome (the previous gold standard). Most importantly, the actual flap thickness is much closer to the thickness labelled on the blade, meaning that surgeons can be more confident about the safety of the flaps they are creating. In addition, the gears are completely covered so that tissue cannot be trapped or jam the mechanism.

4.4.1.2 Moria M2

The Moria M2 is relatively lightweight and compact and enables the surgeon to control flap thickness, flap diameter and hinge length. A detailed nomogram is available to guide choice of equipment for each procedure. The option to use a smaller hinge length means that the stromal bed can be exposed over a greater area for ablation of small eyes or hyperopic corrections; however, a shorter hinge may be more vulnerable to tearing and misalignment of the flap when repositioned. It also allows the hinge to be placed anywhere around the cornea according to the surgeon's choice. Flaps tend to be slightly thicker than stated by the blade. The M2 is also available as a single-use system.

4.4.1.3 Nidek MK-2000

The Nidek MK-2000 is a one-piece microkeratome, in that the suction ring is integral to the microkeratome unit. It therefore does not require assembly on the eye, and the suction time can be reduced. The unit is slightly smaller than others which facilitates placement in eyes with small palpebral apertures. It also tends to cut a flap thinner than stated on the blade. It was designed for creating a nasal hinge.

4.4.1.4 Schwind Carriazo-Pendular

The Carriazo-Pendular has a curved blade and moves across the cornea in a pendular fashion. The cornea is compressed more in the centre than at the periphery, the theory being that this creates a more uniform flap. Flap thickness was highly predictable, even for thin flaps, with standard deviation of 10–12 μm, and flaps tend to be slightly thinner than stated. There is free choice for the location of the hinge. Four suction ring sizes are available and flaps of 9 or 10.5 mm diameter can be created. The hinge can be placed at any location. Flaps can be cut with a thickness of 90–170 μm (20 μm steps).

4.4.1.5 Ziemer Amadeus II

The Amadeus II microkeratome enables the surgeon to choose flap size and thickness as well as hinge length. It can be used as 'three-in-one microkeratome' for traditional Lasik, Epi-Lasik and anterior and posterior lamellar keratoplasty. A nasal hinge is created. It also has variable blade oscillation speed (4,000–20,000 rpm) and translational speed (advance feed rate: 1.5–4 mm/s): faster oscillation creates a smoother stromal bed and faster translation results in a thinner flap. Specific suction rings are required for each flap diameter (8.5–10 mm). The heads (110–160 μm) tend to cut a flap slightly thicker than stated.

4.4.2 Femtosecond Lasers

Femtosecond lasers operate in the near-infrared spectrum (1,053 nm). At low power density, the beam generated is not absorbed by optically clear media. It can however be focussed to a high-power density which is absorbed by the tissue, creating a cavitation sphere within clear media such as the cornea. The power generated is a function of the energy of a pulse and its duration; since power is energy per unit time, the shorter the pulse, the higher is the resultant power of each pulse. The ultra-short pulses delivered by femtosecond lasers (1 fs = 10^{-15}s) are focussed to a spot which is small enough that the fluence (energy/area) is sufficient for plasma formation. The supersonic expansion of the resultant hot plasma creates a tiny sphere followed by a shock-wave and air bubble generation. The combination of these effects disrupts tissue and gives the femtosecond laser its ability to cleave tissues. The precision of this laser derives from the short pulse duration which generates cavitation spheres many orders of magnitude smaller than those resulting from the Nd-YAG laser (≈100 μm).

Current generation lasers use spots of approximately 1 μm, placed by computer-controlled mirrors with an accuracy of approximately 1 μm. The surgeon must program the controller software to create the desired flap diameter and depth and can also decide on the angle at which the side of the flap is formed.

The laser requires that the cornea is contacted by a 'docking plate' for accurate placement of the laser spots; different models have different ways of achieving this.

4.4.2.1 IntraLase FS60 and iFS (AMO)

This was the first femtosecond laser to be used for the creation of LASIK flaps, with the first patient being treated in 2000. The IntraLase FS60 systems are considered 4th generation lasers and have a 60 kHz performance. The current top model, the fifth generation model iFS, operates at 150 kHz and typical energies of 0.8–1.6 μJ (Fig. 4.12). A LASIK flap of 9 mm is created in 8–10 s. Spots can be placed with an accuracy of around 1 μm. The laser unit has a docking system

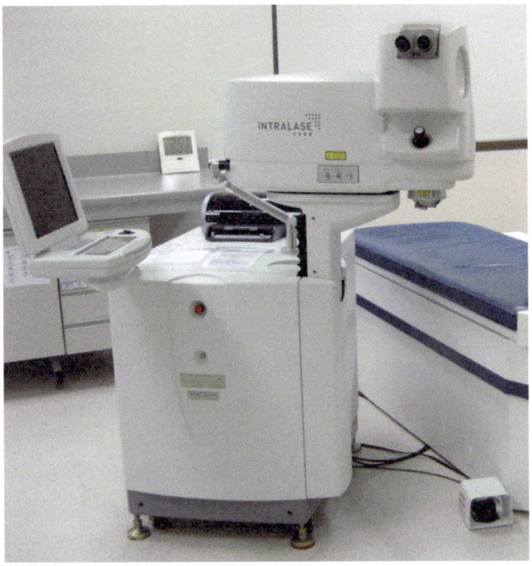

Fig. 4.12 Intralase iFS Femtolaser

with a planar surface so that the cornea is flattened for flap creation.

4.4.2.2 VisuMax (Zeiss)

The laser pulse rate of the VisuMax system is 500 kHz with low energy (0.3 μJ). The typical spot distance is 3–6 μm. A docking system with a concave plate is used so that a curved corneal surface is maintained during flap creation. This represents a more anatomically normal situation and induces less stress within the cornea. This also allows lower suction pressure during flap creation and consequently a lower rise in IOP. It also makes loss of suction less critical during flap creation. The laser beam is automatically centred on the corneal vertex, increasing the accuracy of the treatment. The flap interface is created as a spiral from the periphery towards the centre, allowing the patient to maintain fixation throughout flap creation (compared to raster pattern or centripetal spiral patterns). The unit is very large and requires a large room but is less sensitive to temperature and humidity than other femtosecond laser models.

4.4.2.3 Femto LDV (Ziemer)

The LDV system currently offers the highest frequency (1,000 KHz) and therefore offers the lowest pulse energy (in the nJ range). The laser spots are overlapped so that tissue bridges should become smaller and the flap should be easier to lift. The use of more spots which are smaller, lower energy and more tightly applied may result in smooth stromal beds. The company claims an absence of both inflammation and opaque bubble layer with this model. This model has a focal plane which is fixed during the cut so the geometry available to the surgeon is limited to uniplanar flaps (similar to a conventional microkeratome). The unit is smaller than other femtosecond laser and delivers the laser via a flexible arm assembly which fits under the excimer laser and can be used in a manner analogous to a microkeratome. The advantage of this is that the patient does not need to be moved from one laser to the other.

4.4.2.4 Technolas 520F (Technolas Perfect Vision)

The 520F uses a curved patient interface preserving the normal corneal curvature during the flap creation and therefore reducing the need for high vacuum and patient discomfort. Currently, the laser operates at 80 KHz. The controller software offers the creation of presbyopic Femtolaser treatments (Intracor) and is able to produce corneal flaps and buttons suitable for lamellar and penetrating keratoplasty. It also allows the creation of tunnels for intrastromal ring segment implantation.

4.4.2.5 WaveLight FS200 (Alcon)

The FS200 is a new femtosecond laser for refractive and corneal surgery, operating at 200 KHz and creating a standard 9 mm flap for LASIK in approximately 6–8 s.

Table 4.7 shows a comparison of the advantages and disadvantages of microkeratomes and femtosecond lasers for corneal flap creation in LASIK. There is as yet no strong evidence that either technology is significantly better than the other. Visual outcomes are comparable, although there may be slightly more early haze with the laser flaps. The femtosecond laser may be better for patients with basement membrane dystrophies as there is no shearing force and less risk of epithelial defects.

Table 4.7 Comparison of advantages and disadvantages of microkeratomes and femtosecond lasers for LASIK

	Microkeratome	Femtosecond laser
Advantages	Fast	Low vacuum
	Smooth bed for ablation	Very precise flap thickness
	Flap easy to lift	Thin flaps possible
	No need to move patient between flap creation and ablation	Sidecut profile can be modified to enhance flap stability
	Established technology, lots of experience	Low risk of corneal abrasion
		Less epithelial ingrowth
		Stronger flap adhesion
Disadvantages	High vacuum required generates very high IOP (up to 70 mmHg)	Very expensive
		Bulky equipment
		Longer suction time
	Moving parts may jam during flap creation	Risk of losing suction during flap creation
	Risk of corneal abrasion during flap creation	Tissue bridges must be separated to lift flap
	Risk of button-holes and free caps	Opaque bubble layer may interfere with eye tracker of excimer laser
	Heat generated by blade may affect stromal bed and subsequent accuracy of ablation	Transient light sensitivity syndrome postoperatively
	Fluid brought into interface may make ablation effect unpredictable	Harder to lift flap later if retreatment needed

4.5 Refractive Laser Platforms

The excimer laser used to perform the surgery is guided by computer. The earlier lasers used a broad beam with spot size up to 6 mm to perform the ablation; newer generations use a scanning slit or a 'flying spot' protocol, that is, a small spot (about 1 mm) with many repetitions across the cornea to remove the desired amount of tissue. The broad-beam type used an aperture of varying size to control the size of the beam; the protocol started with a small beam to ablate the centre, and the beam was enlarged to continue the ablation into the periphery. This was limited in accuracy by a central plume of vapour which blocked the beam, resulting in under-treatment centrally and central 'islands'. Scanning slit technology allows a more accurate application of the laser energy and avoids problems with plumes. Flying spot technology further increases accuracy as there is much less interference from plumes, but treatment may take longer. These newer approaches also allow aspheric and wavefront treatment profiles where appropriate.

4.5.1 Alcon Laser Platform (WaveLight)

The current main models are the WaveLight Allegretto Wave Eye-Q and the WaveLight EX500. This laser platform uses a flying spot laser with Gaussian beam profile and a repetition rate of 400 Hz (Eye-Q) and 500 Hz (EX500), which enables an ablation of 1 D in approximately 1.4 s. The spot size is 0.95 mm. The multidimensional eye-tracker samples at 1,050 Hz (EX500) to maintain accurate alignment. This laser also has 'Thermal Optimized Shot Distribution' which is said to help minimise the potential for thermal build-up by better spacing (spatial and temporal) of laser spots.

The Allegretto Wave Eye-Q excimer laser is FDA approved for correction of myopia up to −12 D of sphere with up to 6 D of astigmatism and hypermetropia up to +6 D with up to 5 D of astigmatism with a maximum manifest refraction spherical equivalent of +6.0 D.

Different profiles can be used for ablation, including wavefront-optimised, wavefront-guided, topography-guided, Custom-Q and PTK treatments. Wavefront optimisation (WFO) means that the laser systems perform their ablation with the objective to maintain a natural post-operative corneal shape and thus to preserve the cornea's asphericity. In order to do this, the laser takes the *K*-readings into consideration, adapting each treatment to the patient's individual refraction and corneal curvature.

The Allegretto Wave Eye-Q system comprises a swivelling operating bed, laser beam housing compartment, laser delivery arm, high speed 400 Hz tracker and monitor, integrated slit lamp and portable notebook. The system can also be connected to a separate external monitor and/or recording device. This model also has a relatively small footprint (able to be moved through standard doorways) and is relatively insensitive to temperature and humidity fluctuations (within the ranges of 18–30 °C (65–86 °F) temperature and 20–70 % humidity).

4.5.1.1 WaveLight Analyser

The WaveLight Analyser is a diagnostic device which measures the optics of the eye and calculates the individual wavefront aberrations, needed for wavefront-guided (WFG) treatments as opposed to the standard wavefront-optimised treatment. The rotating panel PC includes both a computer and monitor which can be used for showing patients their individual data.

4.5.1.2 Planning and Programming the Allegretto Wave Eye-Q

Patients will typically have had their preoperative evaluation with or without wavefront assessment carried out prior to the day of surgery. The relevant treatment data is then entered manually into the portable notebook computer. In the case of wavefront-guided treatments, a USB stick is used for the data transfer from the WaveLight Analyser to the Allegretto laser. This can be done on, or before, the day of surgery.

Prior to the surgical treatment, energy and system calibration checks are carried out. Once the laser is ready, the treatment data has been loaded and the corneal surface has been prepared to receive laser ablation (e.g. LASIK flap, epithelial debridement); the patient is asked to fixate on a flashing green light, directly overhead, within a cluster of amber lights. The operating bed has an integrated joystick, which enables precise alignment of the eye to the *x*- and *y*-axis with an accuracy of <0.1 mm. The swivelling speed is adjustable. The bed's power supply is interrupted as soon as the treatment is running in order to prevent unintended bed movements. If the bed is swivelled out, safety is ensured by time-controlled power interruption. Centration along the z-axis is achieved by focussing the two red lights (from target diodes) so that just one is seen, on the corneal surface to be treated. The laser's general illumination setting, patient's palpebral aperture and any fluid/drape reflections may need to be adjusted for, so that the tracker can work effectively.

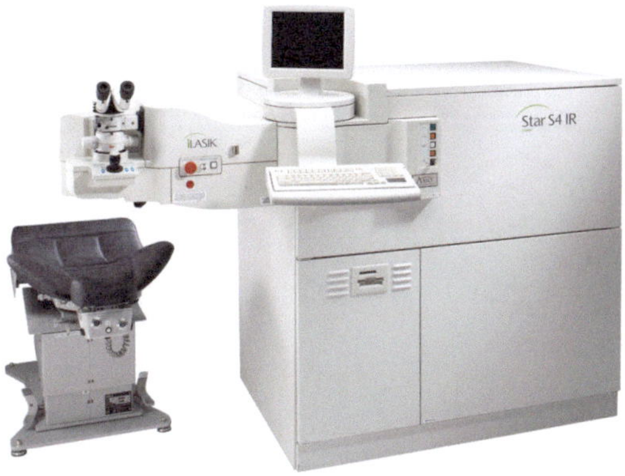

Fig. 4.13 VISX S4 IR excimer laser (Courtesy of AMO)

The surgeon depresses a centration foot pedal to ensure the proposed ablation is centred as desired. The patient continues to fixate on the flashing green light and the surgeon depresses the laser-firing foot pedal. The laser tracker follows the pupil and automatically keeps track of the eye. The laser ablation is completed. The external plume evacuator removes fumes and odours that are created during the laser treatment. A summary of treatment is then printed out for the patient's record.

4.5.2 AMO Laser Platform (VISX)

The current model is the VISX Star S4 IR™ excimer laser (Fig. 4.13). It uses a variable diameter beam of size between 0.65 and 6.5 mm (Variable Spot Scanning, VSS) and effectively combines broad-beam and flying spot technology with variable repetition rates (VRR, 6–20 Hz), depending

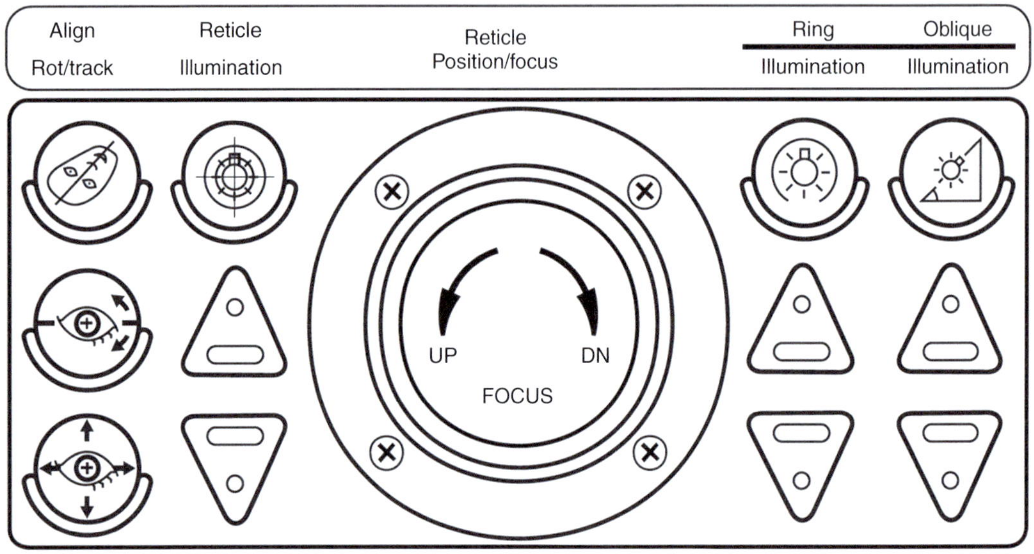

Fig. 4.14 Doctor's keypad

on the size of the spot being applied. The eye tracker offers 3 D active tracking with automatic centring. The iris registration (IR), which locates multiple iris features, provides a high level of alignment accuracy and precision (compensates for cyclotorsional movement), giving the surgeon more confidence that the treatment will be placed in the correct location.

The principle hardware components of the laser system are the doctor's control panel with keypad and joystick (Fig. 4.14), the microscope, a calibration platform and debris-removal nozzle, the patient chair with headrest controls, a laser footswitch, the computer control station with keyboard and the laser gas cabinet. The front control panel features floppy disk and VISX treatment card slots. The doctor's keypad controls the patient alignment via the alignment fiducial, the reticule (Fig. 4.15), the fibre optic ring illumination, the iris registration system and the eye-tracking system.

The VISX S4 laser is FDA approved to treat up to 11 D of myopia, with or without up to 3 D of myopic astigmatism, mixed astigmatism up to 5 D and up to 3 D of hyperopia with or without 2 D of astigmatism.

The WaveScan system (Fig. 4.16) acquires comprehensive wavefront data and takes an image of the patient's eye which is used for iris registration. In combination with the patient's *K*-values, it creates an optimal 'CustomVue' ablation profile.

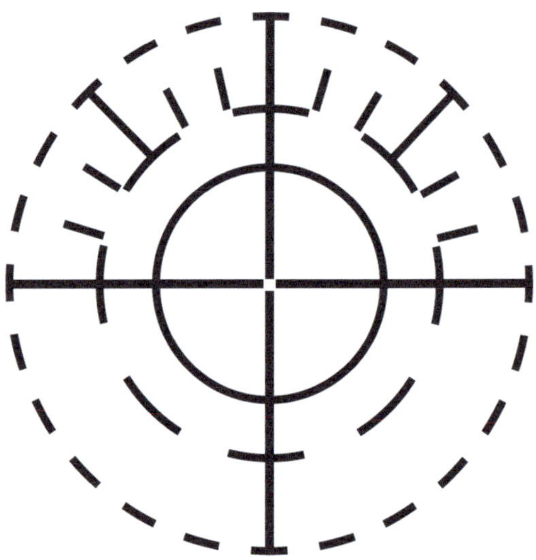

Fig. 4.15 VISX S4 IR Reticule; smallest ring is 4 mm

The CustomVue procedure consists of four steps:

1. Acquisition of wavefront and iris data
2. Review of wavefront scans
3. Planning the treatment
4. Alignment of the eye and treatment

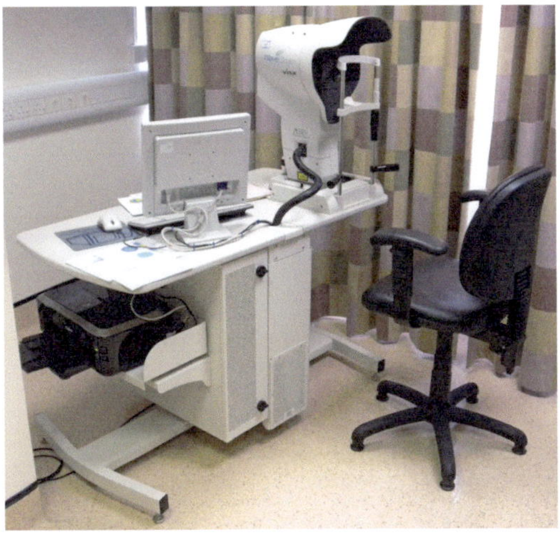

Fig. 4.16 Images of WaveScan aberrometer

4.5.2.1 Acquisition of Wavefront and Iris Data

The use of the WaveScan system starts with a 15-min warm-up period and a verification procedure to check the accuracy of the measurements. Once the accuracy has been verified, new patient data can be entered and saved. The room light is dimmed and the patient is placed properly, with an instruction to look at the fixation target (minimise accommodation by telling the patient to gaze beyond the target). The pupil size should range between 5 and 7.5 mm but must be at least 4 mm (do not use dilating drops). The eye is centred (yellow crosshair and rings in the centre of the pupil) and the focus is adjusted to the inner margin of the iris (for iris imaging). Usually, the autofocus mode is used to focus the Hartmann-Shack image, providing sharply focused circular dots (not oblong in shape). Ask the patient to blink to normalise tear film prior to capture. A minimum of three measurements for each eye with IR ready images (green IR icon/box) should be performed before proceeding to the review process.

4.5.2.2 Review Wavefront Data

At this stage of the procedure, the different scans are reviewed by the surgeon and the best scan is selected for the treatment. Criteria for the selection process include iris focus, scan quality (four green ticks), wavefront cylinder axis matching manifest cylinder axis and wavefront diameter >5 mm.

4.5.2.3 Planning the Treatment

Following the scan selection, further surgical treatment parameters are entered, including the *K*-values (from IOLMaster or autorefractor), preoperative manifest refraction and the central corneal thickness (from ultrasound). The size of the pupil is added from the WaveScan measurement. The doctor then decides on the size of the optical/transition zone. The following basic values can be used and later individually adjusted: for myopia with a normal pupil size, 6/8 mm; for myopia with a large pupil, 6.5/8.5 mm; and for hyperopia, 6/9 mm. The type of laser treatment is entered (e.g. LASIK or LASEK) and individual, nomogram-based treatment adjustments can be performed (experienced surgeons only; e.g. 3–5 % boost in LASEK for young myopes). The treatment ablation profile is then calculated for one eye. The process of treatment planning is repeated for the second eye (it is advised to use the same optical zone for both eyes). A surgical planning form, a surgical treatment plan report (Fig. 4.17) and a custom report (Fig. 4.18) can be printed. Finally, the iris image, wavefront and treatment data are saved on USB flash drive and transferred to the excimer laser (loaded via the E: Drive and use of the refresh button).

4.5.2.4 Alignment of the Eye and Treatment

The first step on the VISX Star S4 IR excimer laser after loading the treatment file is to define the location of the flap hinge (usually superior or nasally), and additional nomogram changes (usually none). Then, the patient is seated on the patient chair and the patient's head is aligned perpendicular to the system with the fiducial line. The cornea is centred in the middle of the interpalpebral fissure (primary position), and the focus is on the corneal surface. The lowest possible level of illumination is used to keep the pupil diameter as close as possible to the WaveScan pupil diameter. In LASIK, the eye-tracker system and iris registration system should be engaged

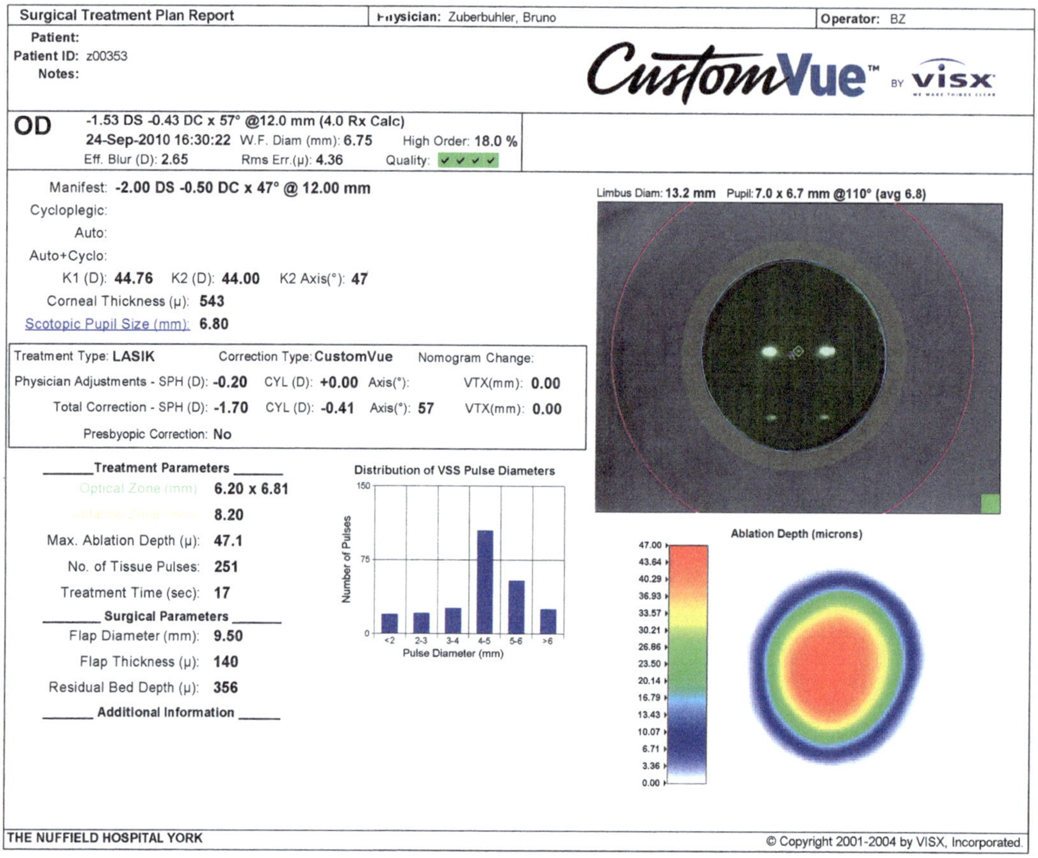

Fig. 4.17 WaveScan surgical treatment plan report

after the flap is elevated. Features of the iris on the WaveScan image are then compared with features located on the image of the iris taken using the excimer laser's camera. The iris registration process is used to align the treatment to the axis of the patient's eye and to correctly centre the treatment independent of pupil centre migration. Once the iris registration has been engaged, the head should not be repositioned again. The foot switch can be pressed to start the treatment once a dialog box has provided the 'OK to treat'. An operative report can be printed at the end (Fig. 4.19).

4.5.3 Technolas Laser Platform

This excimer laser uses a flying spot with spot sizes of 1–2 mm which have a truncated Gaussian beam profile (Fig. 4.20). The pulse frequency is 100 Hz. The six-dimensional dynamic rotational eye-tracking system samples at 240 Hz and uses true iris recognition (about 3,000 points on the iris). The Technolas excimer laser is FDA approved to treat myopia up to −11 D with or without up to −3 D of astigmatism, and hyperopia up to +4 D with or without +2 D of astigmatism.

4.5.3.1 Zyoptix Diagnostic Workstation

This is an integrated diagnostic system for customised refractive treatments, consisting of the Orbscan IIz corneal topographer and the Zywave wavefront analyser (Figs. 4.21, 4.22 and 4.23). The system is networked with the Technolas Z100, allowing direct transfer of patient and treatment data.

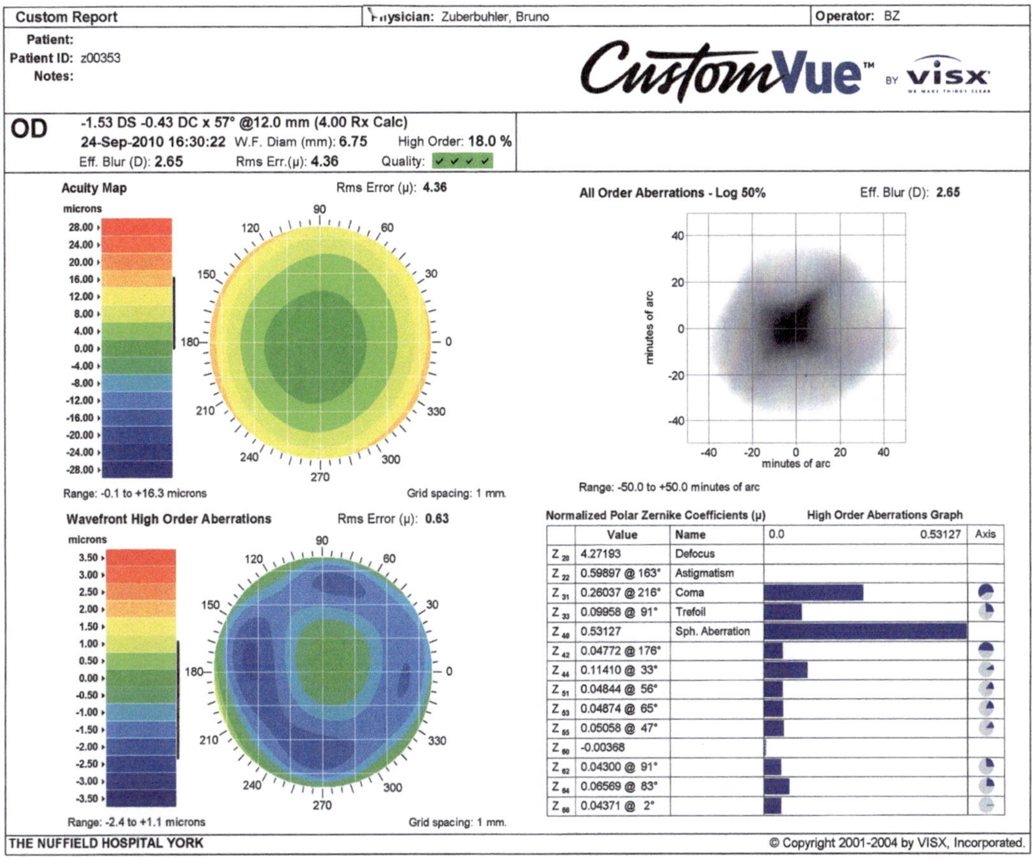

Fig. 4.18 WaveScan custom report

4.5.4 Schwind Laser Platform (Amaris)

The current main models are the Amaris 500E (Fig. 4.24) and the Amaris 750S. The lasers use a 0.54 mm flying spot with super-Gaussian spot profile and a pulse rate of 500 Hz (Amaris 500E) and 750 Hz (Amaris 750S). The active six-dimensional eye-tracker samples at 1,050 Hz, including compensation of linear movements (first and second dimensions), rolling movements (third and fourth dimensions), static and dynamic cyclotorsion (fifth dimension) and movements along the *z*-axis (sixth dimension). The energy fluence level (energy per unit area) is varied through the treatment with high fluence used during the first 80 % of the ablation to reduce the duration of treatment and a lower level used for the last 20 % to maximise precision. Refractive treatments include 'aberration-free' treatment (Fig. 4.25), corneal wavefront, ocular wavefront and presbyopic treatment profiles (PresbyMAX) for PRK, TransPRK, LASEK and LASIK, respectively.

4.5.4.1 Diagnostic Devices

The ocular wavefront analyser is a multifunctional aberrometer, analysing the optical characteristics of the whole eye with a resolution of 230 μm and 1,024 measuring points. The Schwind Sirius (Fig. 1.24) is a high-resolution corneal topographer combining a rotating Scheimpflug camera with a Placido disc, allowing the analysis of the complete corneal wavefront and the topography of the anterior and posterior corneal surface. It offers keratoconus screening tools and pupillometry functions. The 'combi' system enables comparison of corneal and ocular wavefront data.

Operative Report

THE NUFFIELD HOSPITAL YORK Sep 24, 2010 6:13:31PM

Patient Information

ID #: z00
Date of Birth: 9/15/1945
Sex: Male
Referral:

Pre-Op Information

Eye: OD	VA-sc:			VA-cc:
Keratometer:	K1: 44.76 D	K2: 44.00 D		K2 Axis: 47°
Manifest Refraction:	-2.00 DS	-0.50 DC x	47°	12.00 mm
WaveScan® Refraction:	-1.53 DS	-0.43 DC x	57°	12.00 mm
WaveScan® Refraction Pupil Size:	6.75 mm			

Instrument

Facility Name:	THE NUFFIELD HOSPITAL YORK
System Serial Number:	5508
Software Version:	5.22
Target Fluence:	160 mJ/cm²
Transmission:	21.0%
Calibration Table:	0030-4353 Rev.A (-76), STAR S4, CustomVue, International
Calibration Factor:	1.00

Treatment Information (Spectacle Plane)

Procedure:	CustomVue™ Treatment			
Desired Correction:	-1.53 DS	-0.43 DC x	57°	12.00 mm
Physician Adjustment:	-0.20 DS	+0.00 DC		0.00 mm
Nomogram:	0%			
Adjusted Correction:	-1.70 DS	-0.41 DC x	57°	0.00 mm
Optical Zone:	6.8 x 6.2 mm			
Ablation Zone:	8.2 mm			
Exam Date:	24-Sep-2010 09:30:22			
VSS Algorithm Version:	2.367.2006.0926			

Physician Has Specified a LASIK Treatment, Superior Flap

Laser Information (Corneal Plane)

Total Ablation Depth:	47 µm			
Total Number of Pulses:	251 pulses			
Laser Correction:	-1.70 DS	-0.41 DC x	57°	0.00 mm

Treatment Results

Treatment Started:	9/24/2010 6:08:47PM	
Treatment Ended:	9/24/2010 6:10:43PM	Completed
Laser Max Pulse Rate:	20.0 Hz	
Pulses delivered:	251 pulses	
ActiveTrak®:	Enabled, Auto Centering	
Iris Registration:	Enabled, 2.8°Clockwise	

Treatment Center Adjustment(mm): 0.25x, 0.05y.

Notes Information

Surgeon: Bruno Zuberbuhler

Fig. 4.19 VISX S4 operative report

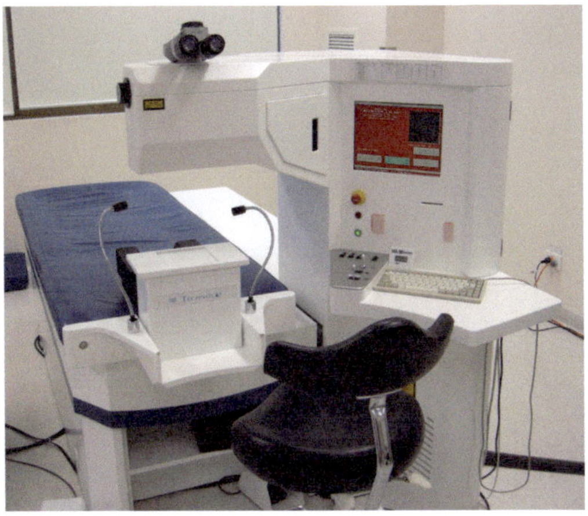

Fig. 4.20 Images of Technolas excimer laser

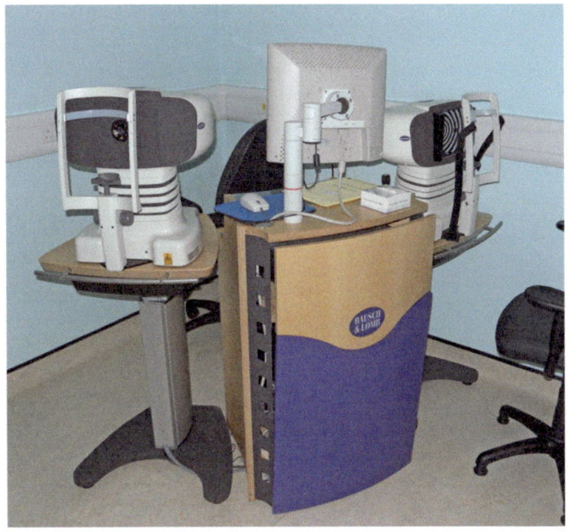

Fig. 4.21 Images of Zywave and Orbscan

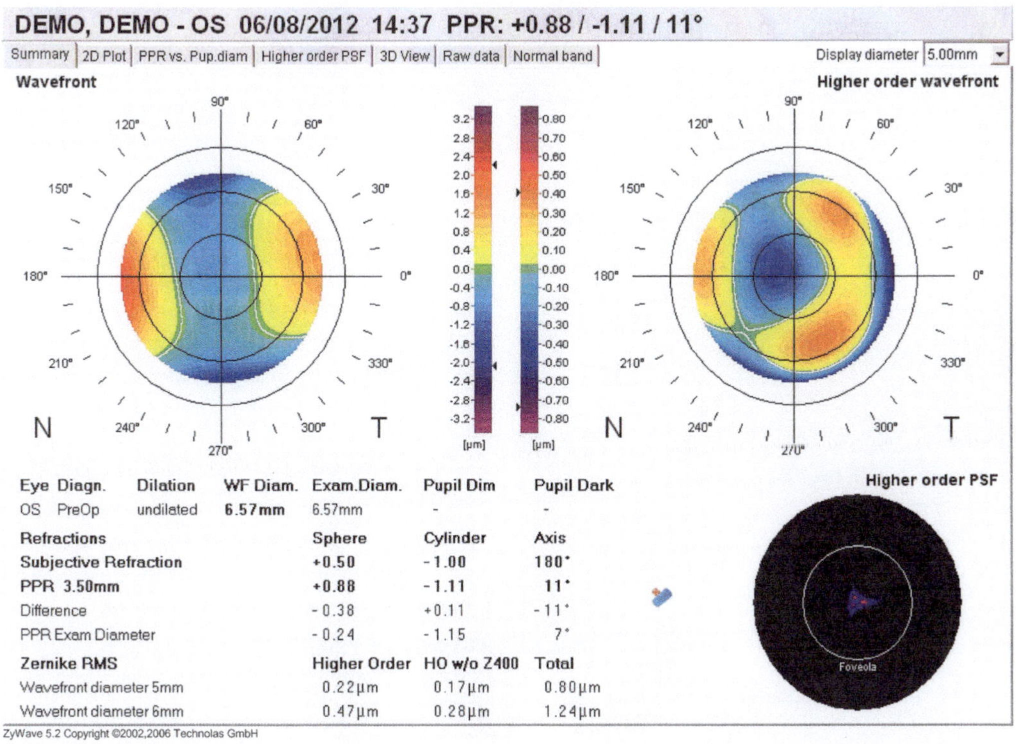

Fig. 4.22 Zywave printout summary

4.5.4.2 CAM Software

This software offers tailor-made treatment planning for a broad application range in refractive and therapeutic corneal laser surgery.

4.5.5 Zeiss Laser Platform (MEL 80)

The MEL 80 uses a flying spot laser with a 0.7 mm Gaussian profile beam and a repeat rate

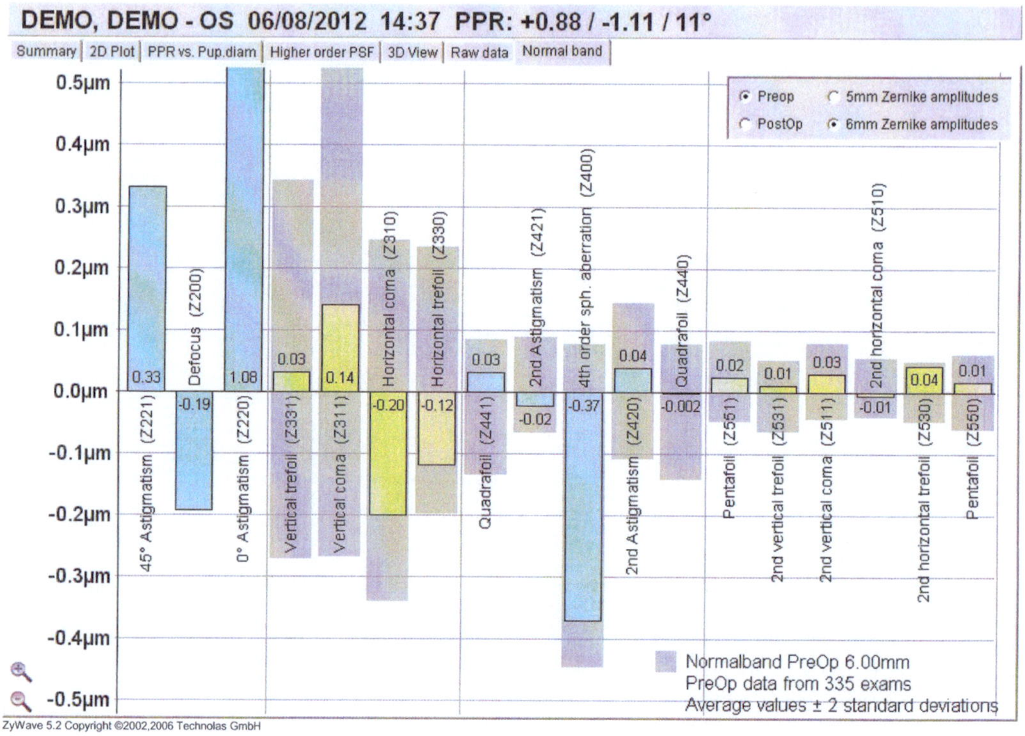

Fig. 4.23 Zywave printout higher-order aberrations

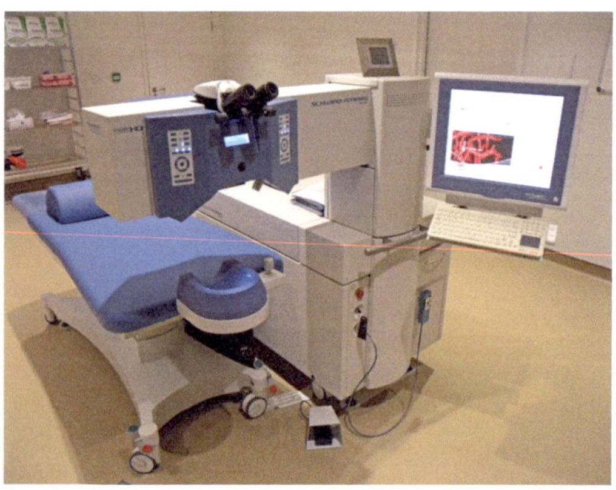

Fig. 4.24 Schwind Amaris 500E excimer laser

of 250 Hz; a correction of 7 D can be completed in approximately 22 s (Fig. 4.26). The eye tracker also samples at 250Hz and there is an option for iris recognition. An atmospheric control system between the laser aperture and the patient's eye creates an airflow which reduces the incidence of beam masking, ensuring accurate ablation. There is a built-in slit lamp which can be useful when lifting a LASIK flap or identifying residual islands of epithelium before surface laser treatments. The laser unit is compact and relatively light which makes it mobile for use in different theatres.

4.5.5.1 CRS-Master

This software and hardware system provides the full spectrum of customised treatment options in combination with the MEL 80 excimer laser. It integrates ocular wavefront (WASCA Analyser) and corneal topography (ATLAS 995) diagnostics into a compact workstation (Fig. 1.26).

4.5.6 Nidek Laser Platform

The current main models are the Quest and the EC-5000CX III. The laser uses a rotating scanning slit to deliver the laser energy with Gaussian profile. Beams of 1–9 mm can be used, with repeat rates of up to 40 Hz. The beam is rectangular and scans, rotates and overlaps to increase the

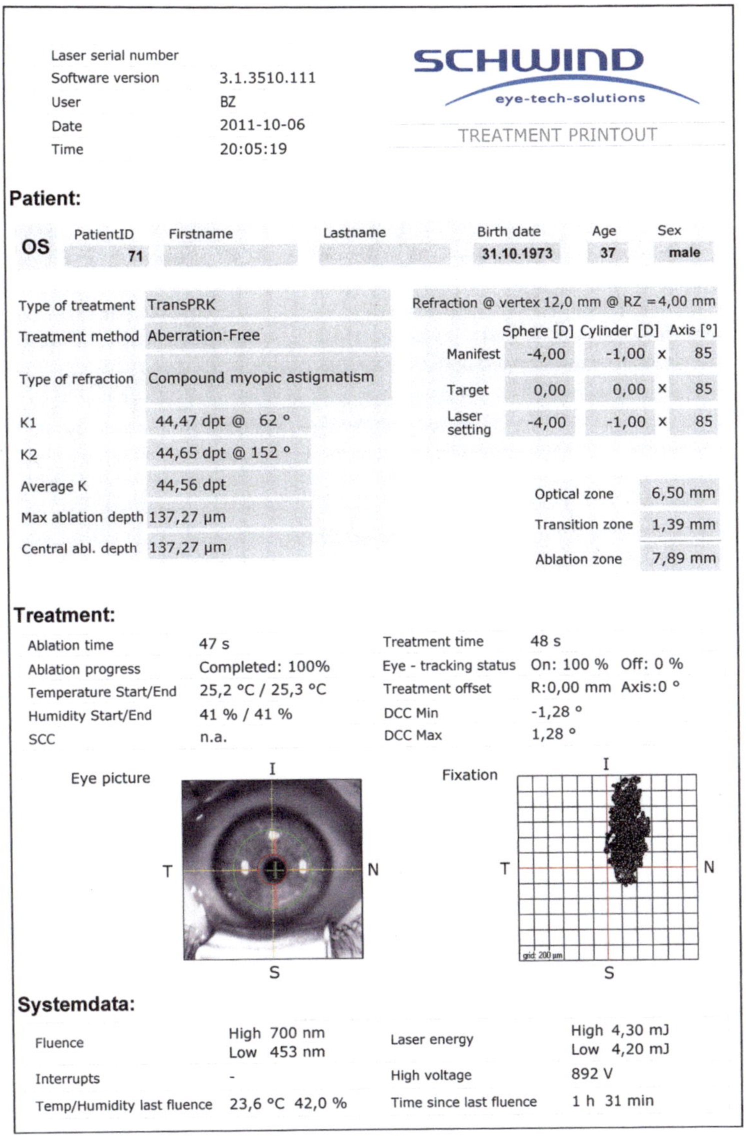

Laser serial number
Software version 3.1.3510.111
User BZ
Date 2011-10-06
Time 20:05:19

SCHWIND
eye-tech-solutions
TREATMENT PRINTOUT

Patient:

	PatientID	Firstname	Lastname	Birth date	Age	Sex
OS	71			31.10.1973	37	male

Type of treatment	TransPRK
Treatment method	Aberration-Free
Type of refraction	Compound myopic astigmatism
K1	44,47 dpt @ 62 °
K2	44,65 dpt @ 152 °
Average K	44,56 dpt
Max ablation depth	137,27 µm
Central abl. depth	137,27 µm

Refraction @ vertex 12,0 mm @ RZ =4,00 mm

	Sphere [D]	Cylinder [D]		Axis [°]
Manifest	-4,00	-1,00	x	85
Target	0,00	0,00	x	85
Laser setting	-4,00	-1,00	x	85

Optical zone	6,50 mm
Transition zone	1,39 mm
Ablation zone	7,89 mm

Treatment:

Ablation time	47 s	Treatment time	48 s
Ablation progress	Completed: 100%	Eye - tracking status	On: 100 % Off: 0 %
Temperature Start/End	25,2 °C / 25,3 °C	Treatment offset	R:0,00 mm Axis:0 °
Humidity Start/End	41 % / 41 %	DCC Min	-1,28 °
SCC	n.a.	DCC Max	1,28 °

Systemdata:

Fluence	High 700 nm Low 453 nm	Laser energy	High 4,30 mJ Low 4,20 mJ
Interrupts	-	High voltage	892 V
Temp/Humidity last fluence	23,6 °C 42,0 %	Time since last fluence	1 h 31 min

Fig. 4.25 Schwind Amaris 500E treatment report

smoothness of treatment. The eye-tracker samples at 200 Hz and uses a torsion error detector (TED) for compensation of cyclotorsion.

4.5.6.1 NAVEX Quest System

This NAVEX System (Nidek Advanced Vision Excimer Laser System) combines the excimer lasers with diagnostic and treatment tools, such as the corneal analyser OPD-Scan III, the OPD-Station software, the custom ablation software Final Fit for wavefront- and topography-guided treatments and the keratome system MK-2000.

4.5.7 iVIS Laser Platform (iRES)

The iRES laser system uses a 0.6 mm dual Gaussian flying spot with a repetition rate of 1,000 Hz. Surgeons utilising the iVIS platform can choose from a variety of treatment strategies, including the advanced surface ablation strategy called cTEN, a one-step, no-touch, trans-epithelial, all-laser-customised refractive treatment. The diagnostic components of this platform include 'pMetrics', for dynamic pupil assessment, and 'Precisio', a high-resolution Scheimpflug-based

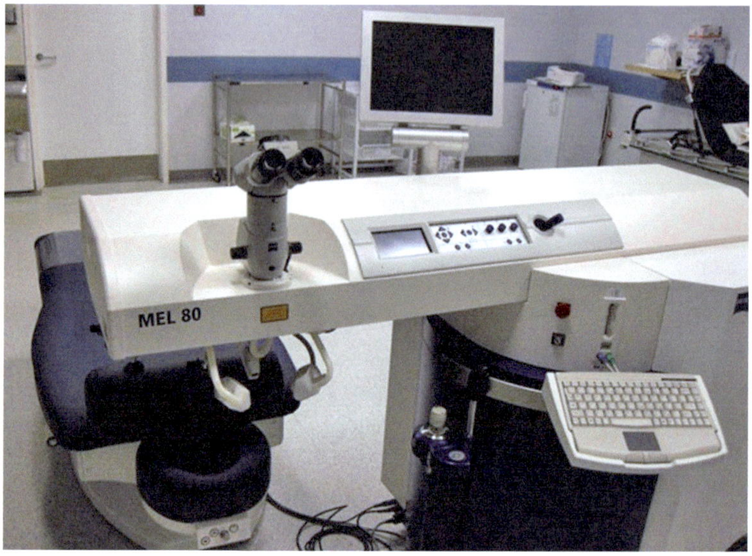

Fig. 4.26 Image of Mel 80 laser; surgeon's view

corneal analyser. An interactive software programme (CIPTA) incorporates a synthesis of refractive, high-definition elevation and pupillometry data into the treatment profile.

4.6 Alternative Procedures

Excimer refractive surgery is not always the best choice, and the surgeon must decide with the patient which procedure best meets their visual needs and expectations. This is particularly relevant as patients become presbyopic or for those who want a reversible procedure.

4.6.1 Clear Lens Extraction (Refractive Lens Exchange, RLE)

This is suitable for patients with refractive errors outside the range treatable with excimer laser refractive surgery (i.e. high myopia >–8 D or hypermetropia >6 D) and for other patients for whom excimer laser is contraindicated.

The surgical procedure is similar to that for small-incision cataract surgery, but as the lens is usually soft, it can be prolapsed into the anterior chamber and aspirated with little ultrasound energy. The surgeon has a wide range of intraocular lenses to choose from, including monofocal (standard or aspheric), toric, multifocal and accommodating. Each lens product has their advantages and disadvantages, and the surgeon must discuss these with the patient.

The benefits of CLE include refractive stability (greater than for excimer laser correction of ametropia) and no risk of corneal ectasia. In addition, studies have shown that the quality of vision with an unoperated cornea exceeds that after corneal surgery because any procedure on the cornea affects the contour and induces optical aberrations. The risks of postoperative complications are also similar to standard cataract surgery and include endophthalmitis, cystoid macular oedema and (particularly for patients with high myopia) retinal detachment, beside others.

4.6.2 Phakic Lenses

Phakic lenses can be placed in the anterior or posterior chamber and have the advantages of preserving accommodation (in pre-presbyopic patients) and being reversible (Table 4.8). A number of different models are available. Some models can be made in toric prescriptions to treat pre-existing corneal astigmatism. The lenses are introduced with forceps (e.g. Verisyse) or injected

Table 4.8 Refractive treatment with phakic intraocular lenses

Location	Product	Complications
Anterior chamber	*Angle supported*:	*Angle supported*:
	AcrySof Cachet (Alcon)	Iritis
	Kelman Duet (Tekia)	Endothelial cell loss
		Pupil ovalisation
		Mis-sizing of haptics
		Glare and haloes
	Iris enclaved:	*Iris enclaved*:
	Artiflex and Artisan (Ophtec)	Slippage of haptics
	Verisyse (AMO)	Erosion at enclavation site
		Endothelial cell loss
Posterior chamber	Implantable collamer lens (Staar)	Cataract formation
	Phakic refractive lens (Zeiss)	Pigment dispersion
		Lens deposits

through a small incision (e.g. ICL), depending on their material. General complications include pupil block, endophthalmitis and refractive surprise. However, complication rates are low and the lenses are usually well tolerated. More details about the surgical techniques can be found in cataract and refractive lens surgery books.

Careful patient selection is important. Table 4.9 shows some accepted inclusion and exclusion criteria (Guell, JCRS 2010).

4.6.3 Intracor

This is a Technolas 520F femtosecond laser-based intrastromal refractive procedure that reshapes the cornea. The laser photodisruption takes about 20 s and creates a pattern with multiple concentric rings in the corneal mid-stroma. The intrastromal cuts lead to a change in corneal power (central steepening). The corneal epithelium and Bowman's layer remain intact. The treatment is used to correct presbyopia for emmetropic or mildly hyperopic patients (+0.75 D) with minimal or no astigmatism.

Table 4.9 Inclusion and exclusion criteria for phakic intraocular lenses

Inclusion criteria	Exclusion criteria
Age >21 years	Active disease in anterior segment
Stable refraction for ≥12 months	Recurrent or chronic uveitis
Ametropia outside treatment criteria for excimer laser correction	Visually significant cataract
Intolerance of spectacles or contact lenses	Ocular hypertension or glaucoma
Iridocorneal angle ≥30°	Autoimmune disorder, atopy, connective tissue disorder, diabetes
Central endothelial cell density >2,500/mm^2 (for age >21 years) or >2,000/mm^2 (for age >40 years)	
Mesopic pupil size <5.0–6.0 mm	

4.6.4 SupraCor

Attempts have been made in the past to incorporate presbyopic corrections into excimer laser ablation profiles to correct distance and near vision simultaneously for the presbyopic patient. Previous treatment algorithms however have encountered difficulties with reduced BCVA due to induced aberrations, particularly spherical aberration and coma. This may be due to creation of the necessary central hyper-positive area.

SupraCor is a novel approach to multifocal LASIK which attempts to implement a presbyopic correction during excimer laser ablation without inducing aberrations within the pupil zone. It is available on the Technolas 217P laser platform (Technolas Perfect Vision) and currently has a CE mark for use in Europe but is not FDA approved and therefore not available in the USA.

Product information claims significant improvement in uncorrected near vision while maintaining good distance vision. Early clinical results from a study involving 46 eyes of 23 patients reported that at 6 months 87 % achieved J2 and

20/25 (near and distance uncorrected acuities) (unpublished data). Patient satisfaction was high and all patients reported being able to function without spectacles.

The inclusion and exclusion criteria for this procedure have yet to be clarified, but it is likely to be most suitable for presbyopic patients with low myopia and little or no corneal astigmatism. Patients with cataract may benefit more from cataract extraction and IOL implant, and this should be assessed carefully before discussing treatment options.

With such as novel procedure, the disadvantages remain to be seen, but as with all attempts to correct presbyopia, this is a compromise between image quality and depth of focus. Consequently, BCVA may not be optimised and contrast sensitivity may be reduced. The procedure is irreversible so thorough patient counselling and a robust informed consent process will be essential. Long-term outcomes are not known and one must consider the possibility that localised epithelial hypertrophy and remodelling may reduce or nullify the refractive effect.

It is also not known yet how the visual outcomes compare with the current alternative procedure, that is, clear lens extraction and multifocal IOL implant.

4.6.5 Conductive Keratoplasty (CK)

This technique remodels the shape of the cornea rather than removing tissue and can be used in the treatment of hyperopia and hyperopic astigmatism and in the management of presbyopia (by inducing monovision).

CK uses radio-frequency energy delivered in a controlled fashion by a fine-needle tip (90 μm diameter) placed into the mid-peripheral stroma to a depth of 500 μm. This results in localised increases in temperature which cause shrinkage of collagen fibrils when the temperature reaches 65 °C. The heat is generated as a consequence of the tissue's resistance to electrical current rather than being directly heated by the probe tip itself. The change induced in the tissue increases the impedance and the current falls, providing a self-limiting effect. This is important as overheating (temperature >70 °C) weakens collagen as cross-links between fibrils are lost and may result in necrosis.

Preoperative assessment includes pachymetry around the treatment zone as well as topography to rule out ectasia, especially keratoconus and pellucid marginal degeneration. Patients with unstable refraction, autoimmune or collagen vascular disorders or who are pregnant or breast-feeding are also excluded from CK treatment. CK may interfere with cardiac pacemakers.

The procedure is performed under topical anaesthesia under the microscope after aseptic preparation and placement of a speculum (no eyelash drape is used as the speculum acts as the return electrode). The patient fixates on the microscope light, while the visual axis and intended location of the treatment spots are marked. Spots are placed in a circle around the 6 mm optical zone (and/or 7 or 8 mm zones) according to the treatment nomogram and depending on the correction required. Each spot delivers 0.6 W at 350 kHz for 0.6 s. Typically eight spots are placed around the circumference of the desired circle. Greater corrections are achieved with smaller treatment zones and more spots. The net effect is to steepen the central cornea. To treat astigmatism, extra spots are placed on the flat meridian. At the end of the procedure, topical antibiotic and steroid eye drops are prescribed.

The refractive results and safety of the procedure were sufficient for FDA approval in 2002 for treatment of hypermetropia of +0.75 D to +3.00 D. There is usually an initial overcorrection (around 0.5 D of myopia) which regresses over the first 3 months. The patient must be warned about a slight compromise to distance vision during the first 3–6 months. The refractive change stabilises between 3 and 12 months after surgery and has been shown to remain stable for at least 3 years. There is probably a degree of regression in the long term due to tissue remodelling and collagen turnover.

Complications reported include foreign body discomfort, transient light sensitivity syndrome and surgically induced astigmatism. The latter can usually be addressed at the initial procedure or as a secondary refinement.

CK is a useful option in the management of presbyopia (correct dominant eye for distance, nondominant eye for near), but patients must be fully counselled regarding monovision and must be motivated to adapt. A contact lens trial is essential.

Success is often greater with CK than with contact lens monovision as the myopia induced in the nondominant eye differs in quality to that with contact lens correction. Patients tend to report less compromise of binocular distance vision, depth perception and contrast sensitivity, perhaps because the treatment enhances depth of field through modifying corneal aberrations. This phenomenon is known as 'blended vision'.

4.6.6 Technique of Femtosecond Lenticule Extraction

As the accuracy and predictability of femtosecond lasers has increased, new procedures for modifying the corneal shape have become possible. These include Femtosecond Lenticule Extraction (FLEx) and Small-Incision Lenticule Extraction (SMILE). Both are performed with the Zeiss VisuMax Femtosecond laser; microkeratome or excimer laser is not required. The spatial accuracy of the Femtosecond laser compared to the excimer laser (i.e. micrometre versus submicrometre) may limit the accuracy of correction of refractive errors with these techniques, but as femtosecond lasers get quicker and spot placement can be made closer, this difference is likely to diminish. This technique has so far only been used to correct myopia with and without astigmatism.

4.6.6.1 Femtosecond Lenticular Extraction (FLEx)

The femtosecond laser is programmed to cut a lenticule within the corneal stroma corresponding to the refractive correction required. The superficial cut which describes the anterior (or external) surface of the lenticule is continued to create a flap (as per LASIK surgery) which is then lifted. The exposed lenticule is removed and the flap replaced. Refractive stability at 12 months appears to be acceptable.

4.6.6.2 Small-Incision Lenticule Extraction (SMILE)

The lenticule is cut using the femtosecond laser as for FLEx, but instead of creating a flap to lift, tunnels 180° apart connecting the lenticule to the peripheral corneal surface are created. Fine forceps can be introduced into one tunnel and the lenticule is grasped and withdrawn from the cornea. The surgeon must ensure that the lenticule is free from surrounding stroma before it is withdrawn by sweeping across both surfaces (anterior, then posterior) with a fine spatula to separate any tissue bridges. After removing the lenticule, the interface is flushed with BSS from one tunnel to the other with a standard LASIK cannula. The tissue planes are created so that the remaining anterior lamella is 110–130 μm thick and its diameter is 7.0–7.5 mm, ensuring that it is 0.5 mm larger than the intended lenticule. The lenticule varies in diameter from 6.0 to 7.0 mm depending on pupil size.

The proposed advantage of SMILE is that as no flap is cut, the structural integrity of the cornea is maintained and the complications associated with flaps are avoided, in particular ectasia, infection, DLK, epithelial ingrowth, flap dislocation and dry eyes. Early data are encouraging regarding safety and accuracy of refractive outcomes. Complications which have so far been reported include dry eye and microstriae (less with SMILE than FLEx) and retained interface debris with SMILE.

After both FLEx and SMILE, the patient is prescribed a regime of topical medication including antibiotic, steroid, lubricant and NSAID eye drops and oral analgesia. Patients are reviewed according to the surgeon's preference, usually on day 1 then at 1 week, 1 month and 6 months after surgery.

The laser parameters for both techniques continue to be optimised to maximise refractive accuracy and to ensure that the surfaces of the lenticules are as smooth as possible to minimise the optical effects of interface healing.

4.6.7 Microwave Thermokeratoplasty (Keraflex)

Also known as Keraflex (Vedera KXS, Avedro Inc.), this is a new technique which uses low-energy microwave pulses to induce local stromal heating (approximately 65 °C) via a dielectrically shielded microwave emitter placed on the epithelium. This leads to collagen shrinkage and formation of a toroidal lesion in the upper 150 μm of the stroma. In the same time, the surface of the cornea is cooled by an evaporative cooling technique to isolate and protect the Bowman's membrane from the thermal effects. This procedure is currently in clinical trials in Europe for the correction of myopia and for the treatment of keratoconus.

The Keraflex procedure differs from conductive keratoplasty (CK) in that in microwave keratoplasty (MK) the electrodes are electrically insulated from the cornea. The energy is derived from interaction between the induced electric field and stromal tissue (i.e. capacitance) rather than a current passing through the tissue as in CK, where heat is generated as a consequence of tissue resistance. The other main difference is that while CK flattens the peripheral cornea and steepens the cornea centrally, MK causes steepening at the site of application and flattening of the central cornea. The difference may be because during MK there is contraction of collagen fibrils in the plane of the fibrils, and there is expansion of the tissue matrix in a direction perpendicular to collagen lamellae. The net result is that the treatment zone acts as a 'spacer' in a manner analogous to intrastromal rings.

The procedure has been used clinically to treat myopia and keratoconus by flattening the central cornea. Topography 1 week after MK for keratoconus showed that irregular astigmatism was reduced and a 'bow-tie' pattern was re-established within a demonstrable treatment zone. Long-term studies will be needed to clarify the stability and duration of this treatment effect. It is possible that the stability of the treatment effect could be enhanced by subsequent cross-linking, either as combined or separate procedures.

An advantage of the Keraflex procedure is that stromal fibres are not cut and the structural integrity of the cornea is likely to be maintained. Long-term studies will be needed to demonstrate this. The epithelium remains intact, reducing the risk of postoperative discomfort, infection and melting. Corneal nerves are not cut so postoperative dry eye is unlikely. Studies also showed that the endothelium was unaffected. However, this technique is in its early development and further work in vitro and in vivo is needed to establish treatment nomograms and treatment limits. Some suggested main exclusion criteria include corneal pachymetry <400 μm, myopic SE of −1.0 D or less, corneas whose K_{max} is centred outside the 4 mm optical zone on corneal topography, history of herpetic eye disease or corneal dystrophy, clinically significant corneal scarring, autoimmune disease, systemic connective tissue disease, atopy, history of chemical injury and if pregnant or breastfeeding.

4.7 Refractive Outcome Analysis (IBRA, Nomograms)

It is essential for refractive surgeons to monitor the postoperative outcomes of their interventions from both visual acuity and refractive perspectives. This helps to refine treatment algorithms in the pursuit of better outcomes as well as identifying any problems. The importance of this should be explained to the patient before surgery to maximise attendance.

A review should be scheduled for 3–6 months postoperative with refraction, topography and wavefront analysis. The data on refractive and visual acuity can be reported in a standard set of graphs (Waring-type graphs; Fig. 4.27). In this way surgeons can monitor their own performance against the profession

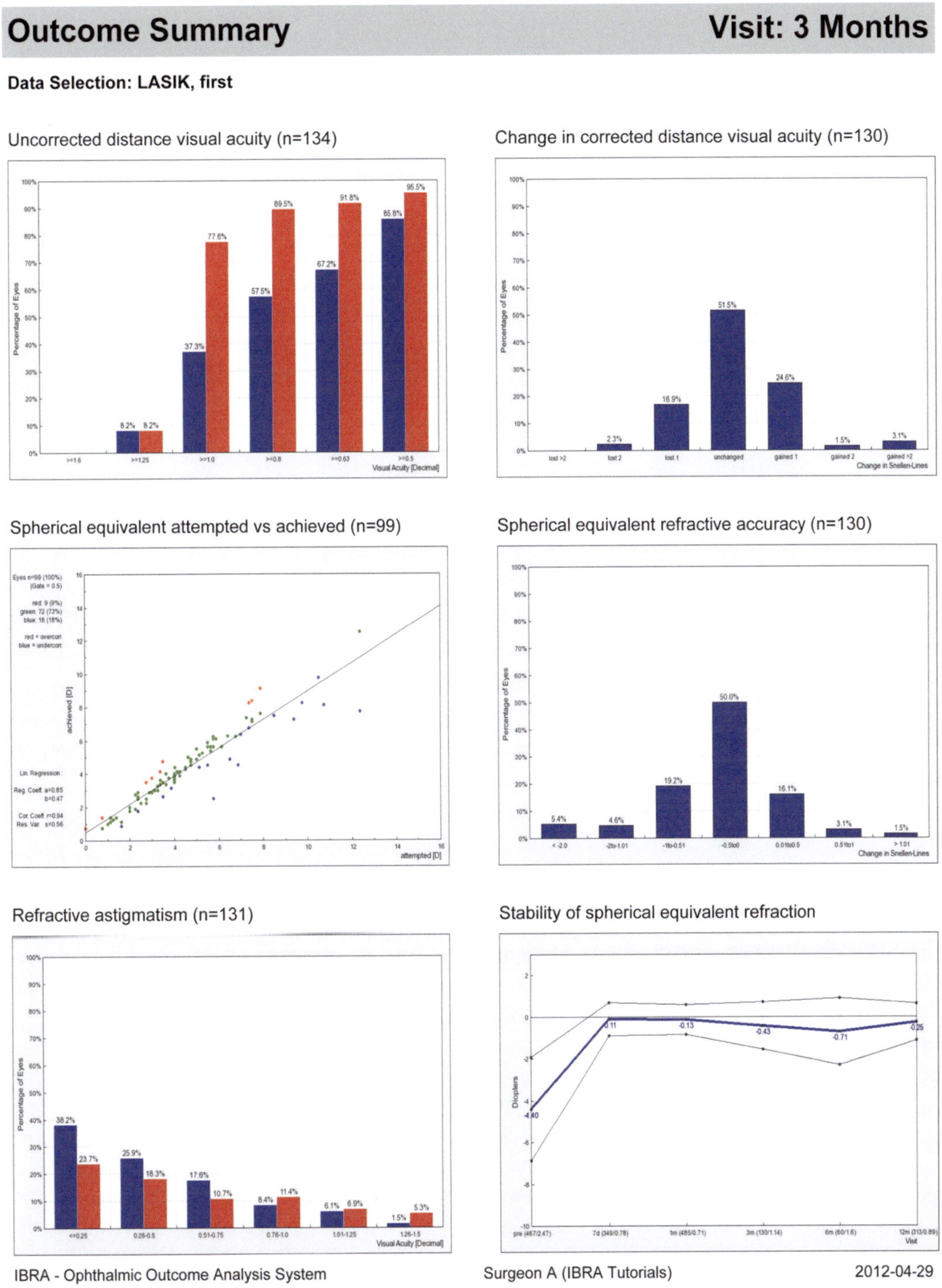

Fig. 4.27 Screenshot of IBRA showing an outcome summary with six charts (Waring type)

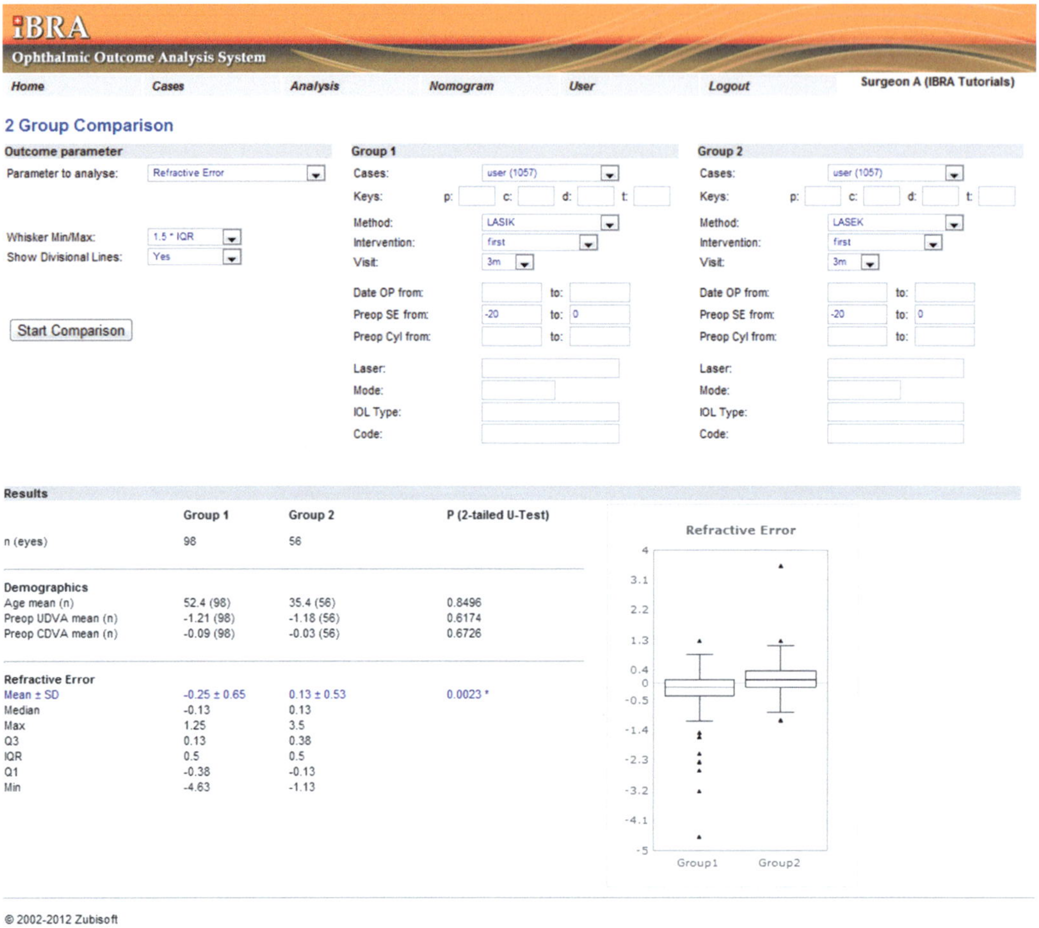

Fig. 4.28 Screenshot of IBRA showing a comparison of LASIK and LASEK treatments

as a whole and outcomes from new techniques can be evaluated.

Specific computer software exists for data collection and interpretation. One of the most sophisticated ophthalmic outcome analysis systems is IBRA (Zubisoft GmbH) with five main focuses: data collection, outcome prediction, outcome analysis (audit), outcome comparison and outcome optimisation. As always, confidentiality with data storage is paramount and measures must be taken to encrypt or anonymise data.

Typical examples of functions, calculations and presentations offered by analysis software:

1. Data collection
   - Sort and show data lists from different treatments, dates of surgery or excimer lasers.
   - Identify outlier graphically or via a comparison with the normal distribution.
   - Undertake multi-centre trials and collect data centrally via a secure Internet connection.
   - Import data from electronic medical record (EMR) systems.

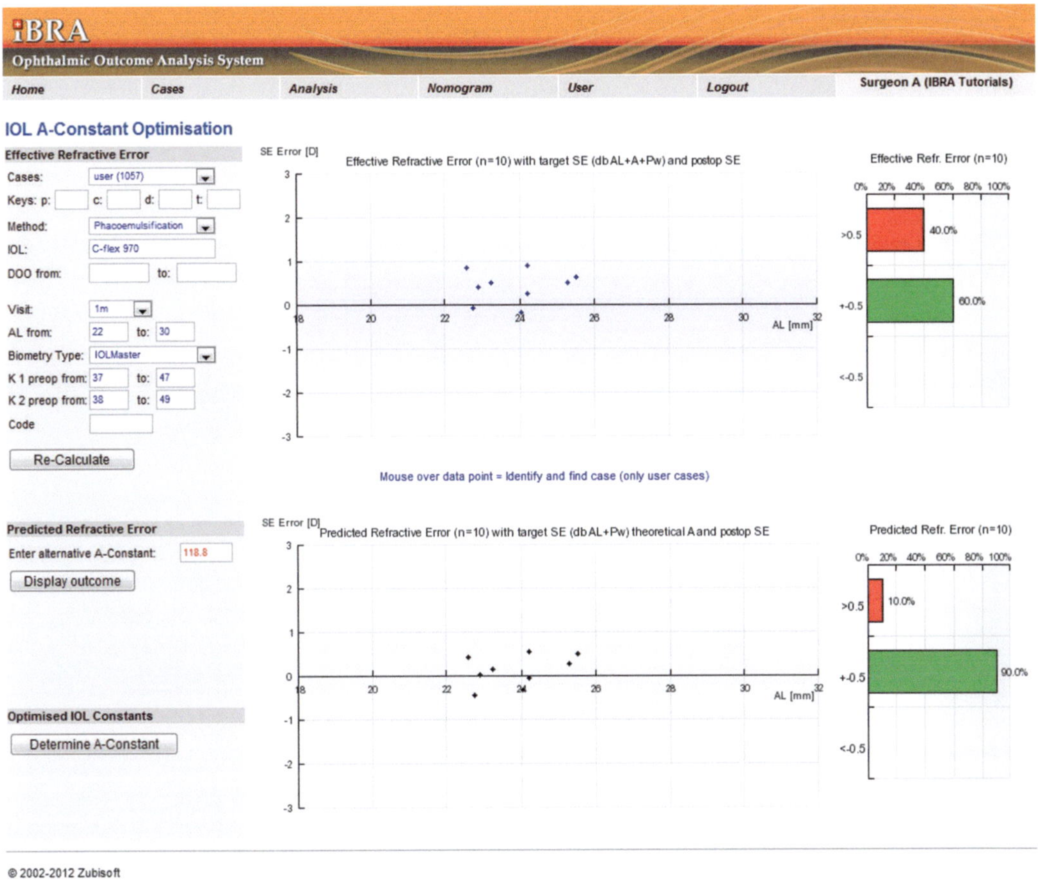

Fig. 4.29 Screenshot of IBRA showing a-constant calculation with outcome forecasting

- Export data to Excel, Minitab or SPSS software for further analysis.

2. Outcome prediction
   - Calculate the chance of spectacle independence for a particular preoperative refraction.
   - Determine the risk of losing CDVA or the need for enhancement treatments after LASIK.
3. Outcome analysis (audit)
   - Present visual and refractive outcomes in accordance to internationally accepted standards.
   - Show the refractive error and outliers after cataract surgery for a particular intraocular lens.
   - Assess induced astigmatism and rotational stability after toric lens implantation.
4. Outcome comparison
   - Compare personal results with a partner, a centre, a group or a reference database.
   - Use statistic tools to calculate differences between data collectives (Fig. 4.28).
5. Outcome optimisation
   - Create treatment nomograms for different refractive groups in LASEK (Fig. 4.29).
   - Calculate the optimised a-constant for a particular intraocular lens (Fig. 4.30).
   - Determine the best intraocular lens power for eyes after refractive laser surgery.

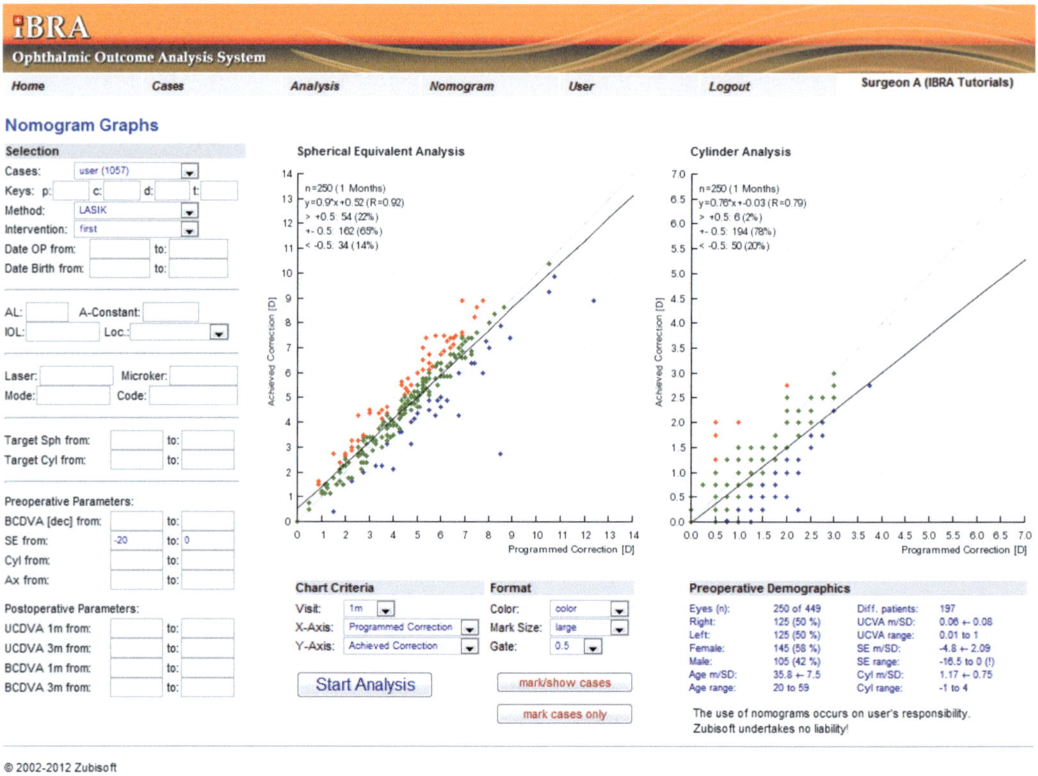

Fig. 4.30 Screenshot of IBRA showing nomogram graphs for myopic LASIK treatments

Wet Lab

5

5.1 Introduction

There has been considerable emphasis in surgical training (as in many other fields) of the importance of simulator-based training in its various forms. Examples which are frequently referred to include those in use in the aviation and space exploration industries, and evidence exists that simulators in medicine are conducive to learning surgical techniques in a safe, patient-free environment. The term 'simulator' in this context refers to wet lab facilities as well as computer-based resources.

Competence in practical skills can only be gained by repeated conscientious practice. It is estimated that mastery of any skill (musical instrument, sports, etc.) requires around 10,000 h of experience and in surgery this is only really possible if a practice environment is available. In the USA, access to a wet lab is a prerequisite for training programmes in ophthalmology; in the UK this requirement is less explicit.

A wet lab is a facility for learning surgical techniques in a safe, patient-free environment. Traditionally, this has involved the use of artificial materials as well as animal or human tissues. Surgeons are able to practice manoeuvres repeatedly until competence is gained.

In ophthalmology in general, this has been used for some time in learning cataract surgery. In corneal surgery examples could include:

- Corneal suturing, corneal trephination and graft suturing
- Flieringa ring suturing
- Creating corneal tunnel incisions
- Lamellar dissections
- Descemet's membrane stripping
- Corneal gluing
- Amniotic membrane grafting
- Intrastromal ring implantation
- LASIK flap creation

If animal tissue (e.g. pig eyes) is used, there should be a formal agreement with an approved source and tissue must be disposed of by incineration after use. It is essential that precautions are in place to ensure that animal tissue is kept completely away from any patient environment (especially operating theatre) and that there is no chance of equipment being transferred between wet lab and theatre. This removes any potential for exposure of patients to microorganisms or prions present in animal tissue.

5.2 Wet Lab Requirements and Maintenance

Six key components have been proposed to the successful establishment and maintenance of a high-quality wet lab:

1. Setting up the physical space
2. Establishing appropriate teachers and curriculum
3. Obtaining the practice eye

B. Zuberbuhler et al., *Corneal Surgery*,
DOI 10.1007/978-3-642-12502-7_5, © Springer-Verlag Berlin Heidelberg 2013

4. Stabilising the eye
5. Preparing the eye
6. Funding the facility

5.2.1 Physical Space

A dedicated area must be assigned for the wet lab which is purely for teaching and practice and not for human surgery (Fig. 5.1). The wet lab should be of sufficient space that several people can work comfortably. There should ideally be several workspaces with ergonomically appropriate seating and adequate lighting. There must be room for the microscopes, ideally one per workstation, together with their controls. The optimal arrangement for this would be to have foot-pedal controls to most closely recreate the operating theatre setup. Microscopes should have a teaching arm so that the trainer can observe with a stereoscopic view. Some larger wet labs also have cameras mounted on each workstation linked to a central computer display so one trainer can switch between views or project one camera feed onto a large presentation display.

There must also be a sink and water supply and enough power outlets to meet the demand safely. The room should have sufficient storage for all the equipment and consumables (Figs. 5.2, 5.3 and 5.4). If cataract surgery is to be taught, there must also be room for the phacoemulsification equipment. If animal eyes are to be used, a fridge to store them in is essential. Appropriate provision must be made for disposal of tissues, sharps and other items.

The facility will require ongoing maintenance and cleaning, and the consumable items will need to be restocked periodically. This is more likely to be carried out satisfactorily if one or more permanent staff take on this responsibility. Users should document their time in the wet lab, primarily for their own training record but also to demonstrate that the facility is being used. Users should also be encouraged to clean after themselves and leave the equipment ready for the next user.

5.2.2 Establishing Appropriate Teachers and Curriculum

It is said that 'practice makes perfect'. However, this is not absolutely true – only *perfect practice* makes perfect. It is vital that trainees have the opportunity to be taught and supervised in the wet lab, or they may develop bad habits. Unskilled trainees using the facility are more likely to damage equipment or, at the very least, make inefficient use of their time unless experienced and willing teachers are available.

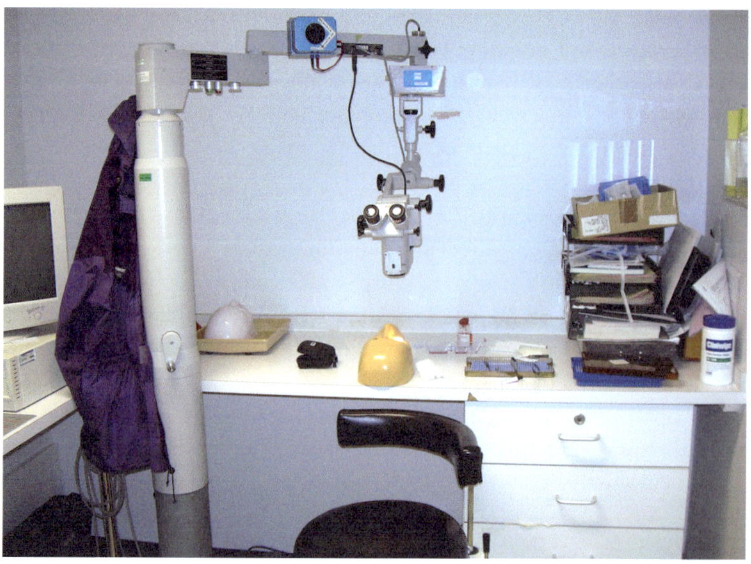

Fig. 5.1 Wet lab setup with microscope and space for instruments

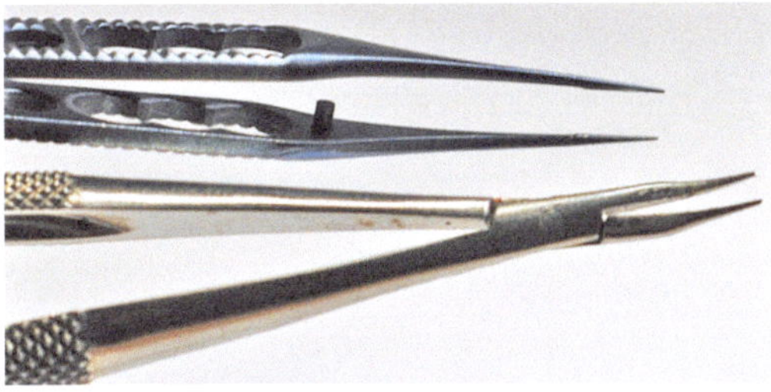

Fig. 5.2 Needle holder and tying forceps (minimal instrument set for keratoplasty practice)

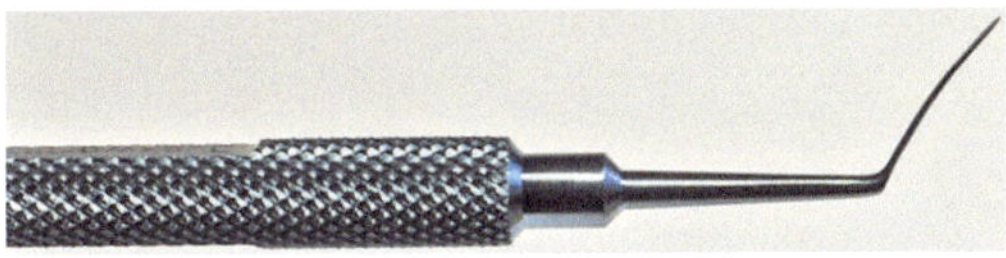

Fig. 5.3 Morlet lamellar dissector (for DALK practice)

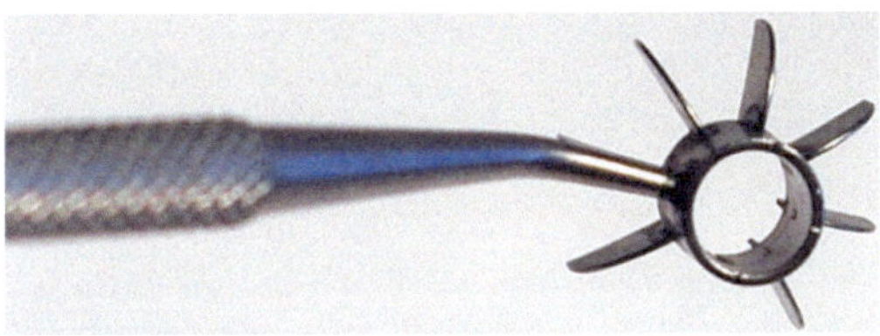

Fig. 5.4 Corneal marker with blade defect (can be used in the wet lab for keratoplasty)

This is difficult to arrange on a regular basis but will greatly enhance the learning experience, and trainees are more likely to progress rapidly if taught well. It is likely in a large department that one or more consultants will have sufficient interest in training juniors to organise a system in which trainees have regular or semi-regular supervised access to the wet lab, at least during the early stages of their surgical training.

For some aspects of training, it may be appropriate for a senior trainee (e.g. a cataract or corneal fellow) to supervise juniors in the wet lab; this is beneficial to both parties as senior trainees are often also called upon to supervise junior trainees in live surgery. This can be quite stressful to start with and the opportunity to have had a 'practice run' in a risk-free environment can reduce the stress involved during actual surgery.

A schedule should be drawn up regarding skills and exercises to be completed in the wet lab before a trainee is permitted to operate on patients.

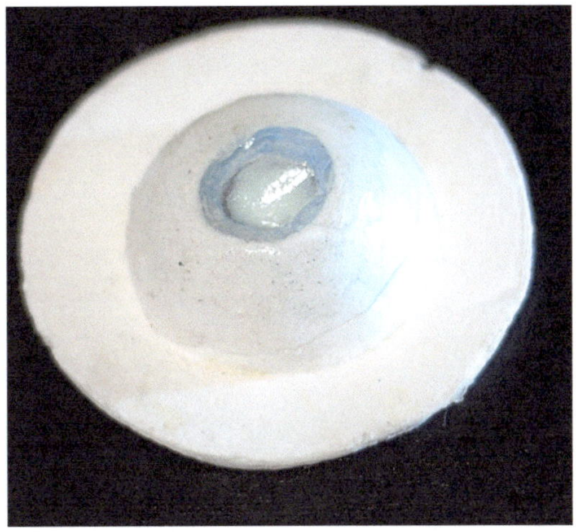

Fig. 5.5 Artificial eye (plastic)

In the UK, the Royal College of Ophthalmologists requires all trainees starting ophthalmic specialist training to attend a Basic Microsurgical Skills course at the beginning of their training which must be completed satisfactorily before they are permitted to operate on patients. This gives trainees an understanding of what types of skills they will require during their training and the level of competence which is expected.

5.2.3 Obtaining Practice Material

There are a number of sources from which mate rial for use in the wet lab can be obtained.

5.2.3.1 Plastic Eyes

Several companies market prosthetic eyes and phantom heads which have traditionally been used in practicing steps of cataract surgery but can also be used in practicing some aspects of corneal surgery (Figs. 5.5 and 5.6). The Royal College of Ophthalmologists is able to supply both eyes and mounts in the UK. These are easy to obtain and clean to work with. However, the handling characteristics are quite different to human tissue, and they can be expensive.

5.2.3.2 Animal Eyes (Especially Porcine)

Porcine eyes have long been used in ophthalmic surgery training as they are widely available and

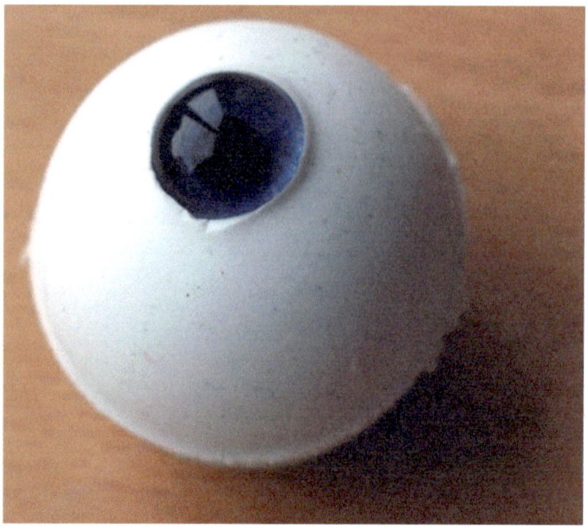

Fig. 5.6 Artificial eye (plastic) from Pharmabotics Ltd

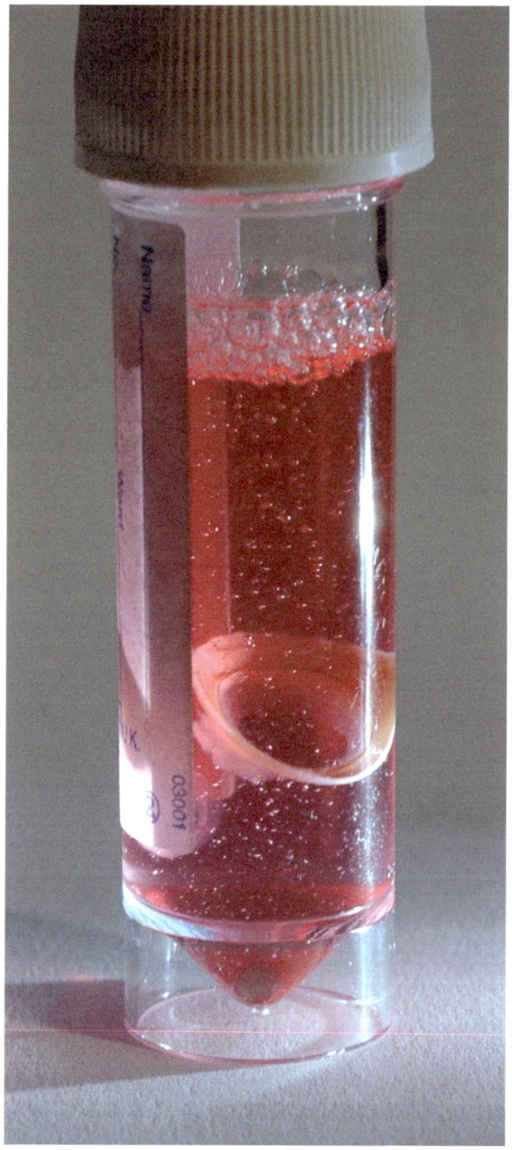

Fig. 5.7 Corneal graft material in bottle

inexpensive to obtain. There have been some concerns recently over the risk of transmission of infective agents to wet lab personnel and trainees, but this has not been reported in the literature. The tissues behave quite differently to human tissues (thicker cornea, elastic capsule) so trainees must exercise caution when progressing to surgery in the operating theatre.

5.2.3.3 Human Corneo-Scleral Discs

Donated human tissue deemed unsuitable for transplant can sometimes be sourced from eye banks. Proper procedures must be in place for the transfer and disposal of tissue, and the original consent must be valid for training purposes. This is the most lifelike way of practicing corneal surgery, but supply of tissue is unpredictable. The disc (Figs. 5.7 and 5.8) can be mounted on an artificial anterior chamber (as used for preparing an endothelial graft), and a range of skills can be practiced (suturing lacerations, lamellar dissection, etc.).

5.2.4 Stabilising the Eye

The ideal mount will closely replicate surgery in terms of eye position, tension, stability, response to surgeon manipulation and ease of positioning under the microscope.

The mount chosen to stabilise the eye will depend on the material being used. Plastic eyes can be mounted in the mannequin marketed for the purpose, a surgical skill board (Fig. 5.9) or a home-made alternative (e.g. adapted wigmaker's dummy head). This will hold the plastic eye securely but there will be no movement in response to manoeuvres by the operator.

Custom-manufactured devices incorporating suction fixation of the eye are available (e.g. Mandell eye mount). One device was described which combined the ergonomics of a polystyrene phantom head and a suction mount.

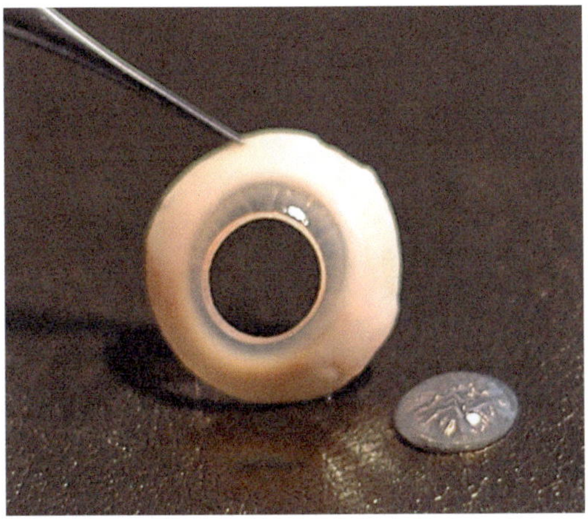

Fig. 5.8 Corneal button and corneo-scleral ring (human)

In the description, suction was provided by the wall-mounted suction system in the operating theatre. This facility may not be available in all wet labs but may be replicated with a large-enough syringe and a pinch clamp on the connecting tubing. By adjusting the suction, the intraocular pressure could be varied to replicate a range of surgical situations.

A more complex device incorporates a red reflex and allows simulation of a range of anterior segment surgical procedures as well as YAG laser iridotomy. This is however more complicated and time-consuming to set up.

Human corneo-scleral discs can be mounted on an artificial anterior chamber which lacks the ergonomics of a phantom head but allows close control of simulated intraocular pressure via a syringe of air, balanced salt solution or viscoelastic and a pinch clamp.

5.2.5 Preparing the Eye

Plastic eyes require little setting up and can be used straight from the box. Some versions are supplied with a flat anterior chamber which must be filled with viscoelastic to reform the anterior chamber. The eye is simply placed in the mount and secured.

Porcine eyes should be reinflated to the required tension by injecting balanced salt or normal saline via a 30G needle through the optic nerve stump or obliquely through the sclera into the vitreous cavity. This may need to be repeated during practice if the eye deflates.

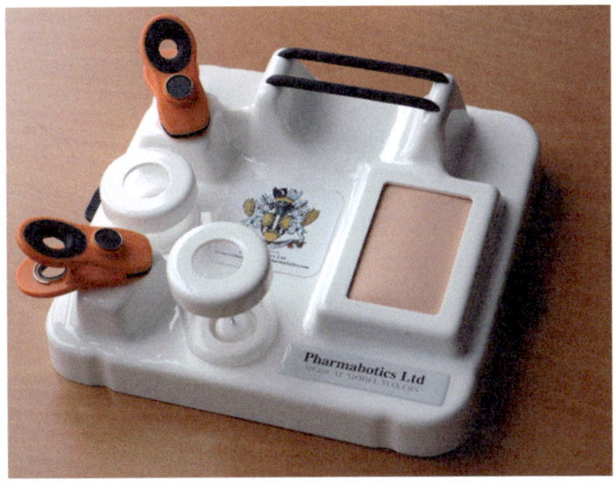

Fig. 5.9 Surgical skill board (Pharmabiotics Ltd)

Human corneo-scleral discs (Figs. 5.7 and 5.8) may be supplied in dextran or the more inexpensive tissue culture medium. Dextran is very expensive but the cornea will be clear as the solution is osmotically optimised. Corneas transported in organ culture undergo osmotic swelling and become cloudy; they can be immersed in dextran or suitable alternative to de-swell them, but this takes several hours, so advanced planning is required. Alternatively, the epithelium can be removed and the corneal oedema reversed by placing glycerol on the surface.

5.2.6 Funding the Wet Lab

The challenge of acquiring sufficient funding to establish *and* maintain a high-quality wet lab should not be underestimated, especially in a difficult economic climate. However, with thought and commitment, this should be achievable, particularly as trainees with access to wet lab facilities are likely to learn faster and encounter fewer complications when they undertake surgery on patients.

Once the profile of the wet lab within the department becomes established, it may be accepted that funds be allocated specifically to the wet lab from the 'training budget' to ensure that it remains a useful resource. Alternative sources of funding might be via industry donations or charitable donations. Consumables (e.g. gloves, viscoelastic devices, intraocular lenses) which have expired and cannot be used in surgery anymore might be passed to the wet lab. Research grants to conduct studies in the wet lab might be available, and publication of research will raise the profile of the facility. Courses (with fees) could be offered on specialist techniques to interested trainees and specialists from further afield which would generate income.

Again, it is preferable that a single individual should take financial responsibility for the wet lab budget and good quality accounts should be kept and made available if required.

5.2.7 Wet Lab Etiquette

If all users of the wet lab take care in their use of the facility it is likely to remain in good order and easy to use. Some facility rules might include:

1. Be considerate to other users; take it in turns if space is limited and do not disrupt others (e.g. music, loud chatter). In a busy unit a booking system may be helpful.
2. Continue collecting consumables (i.e. discards from operating theatres, sample instruments from manufacturers); if all users contribute, stocks are more likely to be maintained.
3. Look after the equipment. If you do not know how to use something or where it goes, ask for advice.
4. Clean up after yourself. Arrange disposal of sharps and animal tissues appropriately.
5. Leave the facility in the state you would wish to find it in.

5.3 Corneal Wet Lab

The following subsections provide examples of corneal surgical techniques that can be practiced in the wet lab.

5.3.1 Corneal Punch

Set out the appropriate corneal punch on the workspace (Fig. 3.12). Ink marks can be applied to the vacuum holes to aid centration if desired. If a human corneo-scleral disc is used, place it epithelium-down on the punch. If a pig cornea is used, first excise a corneo-scleral disc from the whole eye and then place this on the punch. If a vacuum punch is used, squeeze the plunger on the syringe before placing tissue on the block. Use the tissue compression ring to secure the tissue onto the block and release the plunger to apply the suction. The trephine can then be fitted. Press down firmly to cut the tissue – you should feel a 'crunching sensation'. If a pig cornea is used, more pressure will be required than for a human cornea. Press down at each corner to ensure a clean cut. Remove the trephine and dispose of in a sharps bin. Remove the rim and put to one side. Release the suction and remove the trephined disc.

The disc and its rim can then be used in suturing practice to simulate suturing a penetrating keratoplasty.

5.3.2 Lamellar Dissection

Place the corneo-scleral disc on the artificial anterior chamber (Fig. 3.16) and apply the locking ring. Using an air-filled syringe, fill the device with air to the required tension and apply the pinch clamp. The system should not be over-pressurised as this will make dissection difficult. Mark the centre of the cornea and an 8 mm circle around this with a surgical marker pen (a freehand trephine marked with ink can be used for this). In the periphery of the cornea, make a tangential incision with a guarded depth blade (e.g. 350 μm (for DSEK) or 550 μm (for DALK) according to personal preference). A set of lamellar blades is needed to start the dissection.

For DSEK preparation, use the shortest lamellar blade to start the lamellar dissection, taking care to stay in a plane parallel to the corneal surface rather than directing the dissection anteriorly or posteriorly (which would perforate Descemet's membrane). Once a plane has been started, a semi-sharp blade (e.g. Morlet lamellar dissector, Fig. 5.3) is used to continue the dissection across the whole of the cornea, extending to the corneal periphery. Take care to stay in the same plane – this will require rolling the blade to each side of the midline and lifting the heel of the blade once the tip is past the centre to avoid cutting too closely to the epithelium. Once the lamellar dissection is complete, the tissue can be removed from the artificial anterior chamber and an 8 mm graft punched out as above. The lamellae can be separated and inspected for thickness and uniformity. If anterior segment OCT is available, it may be possible to measure thickness.

Practice the technique of introducing the graft into the eye, for example, loading the graft into a DSEK glide if available.

For practicing DALK, start the lamellar dissection as above but identify the reflection of the blade tip. Aim to dissect in the pre-Descemet's plane so that remaining stroma is minimised; this can be judged by having the tip and its reflection as close as possible without them touching. Maintain this as the dissection proceeds. Change to the medium blade once into mid-peripheral stroma and the longest blade once past the corneal centre. Continue the dissection just outside the proposed diameter of the graft so that the host stroma is undermined for suture placement. Once the dissection is complete, inject viscoelastic into the interface to separate the layers. Use a vacuum trephine to remove the anterior stroma; once the trephine cuts through and viscoelastic is seen, release vacuum and remove the trephine. Complete the trephine with curved scissors. Remove the anterior stroma and inspect the bed. There should be little remaining stroma; careful hydration and dissection of this may allow exposure of bare Descemet's membrane.

There is then an opportunity to practice suturing the 'graft' (i.e. the piece of tissue you just removed) back into the rim. The undermined edge of the rim allows deep suture placement without risking perforation of DM.

It is also possible to practice DALK preparation by the big-bubble technique – mount the tissue as before but fill the artificial anterior chamber with saline or BSS. Mark the centre of the cornea and the desired graft size. Using a vacuum trephine cut down into cornea to around 1/3 to 1/2 thickness. Insert a 27G needle on a syringe of air at the base of this cut into mid-peripheral stroma, keeping the bevel down and aiming to place the needle tip in deep stroma. Inject air and observe for formation of a big bubble. If a bubble is seen, withdraw the needle and dissect off a lamella of anterior stroma. Decompress the anterior chamber slightly and using a fine blade make a nick into the bubble in an upward sweep. This should create an opening via which viscoelastic can be injected to open the space between DM and stroma. The remaining stroma can then be cleared with Vannas scissors leaving bared DM.

5.3.3 Corneal Suturing

Various wet lab mounts can be used to practice corneal suturing, the simplest being a plastic eye with a full-thickness cut through the cornea. It is also simple to prepare a pig eye for this by mounting it and making a full-thickness incision. The trainee is then observed in their approach and technique of repair. In true trauma cases, there may be irregular, shelving or stellate lacerations, and opportunities should be created to practice repairing all of these.

In practising corneal graft suturing, the trainee should concentrate on alignment, depth, length and tension of sutures (Fig. 1.7). Interrupted and continuous sutures can both be practiced (Figs. 5.10, 5.11 and 5.12). The trainee must keep the mounted eye still and move their hands around as per live surgery rather than cheating by turning the eye round so that suturing is easier!

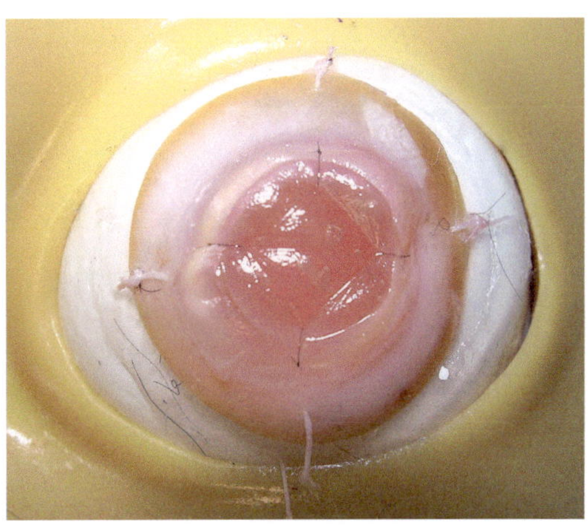

Fig. 5.10 Keratoplasty in the wet lab: four cardinal sutures form diamond-shaped tension lines

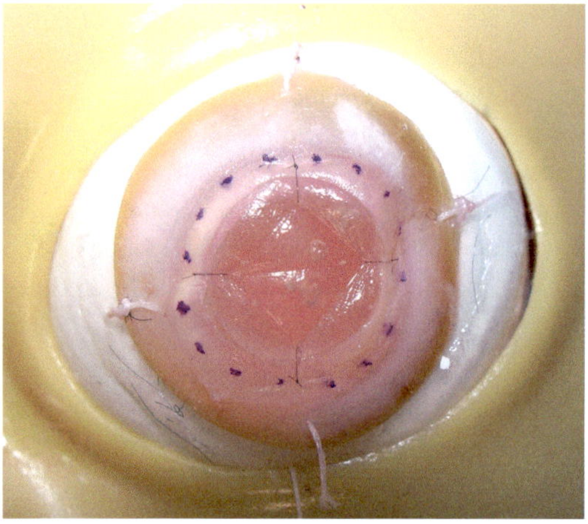

Fig. 5.11 Keratoplasty in the wet lab: 16 marks on the host cornea for a running suture

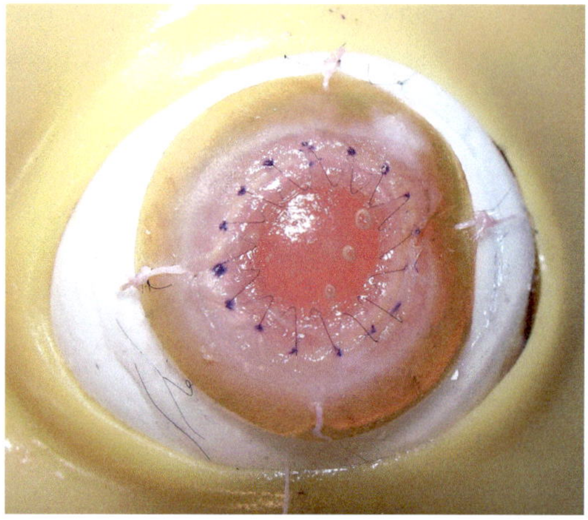

Fig. 5.12 Keratoplasty in the wet lab: suture adjustments and tensioning

5.3.4 Flap Creation

This is only practical on tissue (i.e. porcine or human) rather than plastic eyes. The eye is mounted in the usual way and the suction ring is applied. It may be difficult to achieve adequate suction with a pig eye due to the differences in corneal curvature and diameter, particularly if the intraocular pressure is low to start with. It may be necessary to inflate the eye with saline before starting. The trainee can practice mounting the microkeratome and making the forward and reverse passes. Once the assembly is removed, the trainee can practice lifting and replacing the flap.

Index

B. Zuberbuhler et al., *Corneal Surgery*,
DOI 10.1007/978-3-642-12502-7, © Springer-Verlag Berlin Heidelberg 2013

MIX
Papier aus verantwortungsvollen Quellen
Paper from responsible sources
FSC® C105338

If you have any concerns about our products,
you can contact us on
ProductSafety@springernature.com

In case Publisher is established outside the EU,
the EU authorized representative is:
Springer Nature Customer Service Center GmbH
Europaplatz 3, 69115 Heidelberg, Germany

Printed by Libri Plureos GmbH
in Hamburg, Germany